THE PICTURE BOOK OF
TRAINS

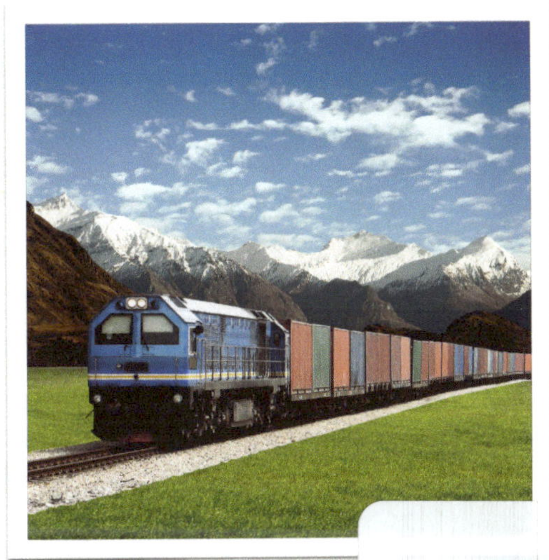

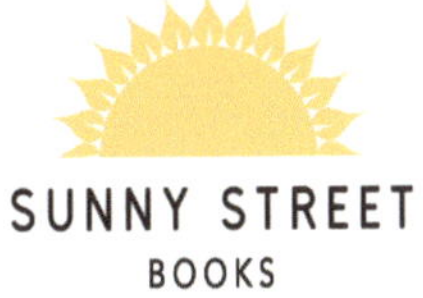

SUNNY STREET
BOOKS

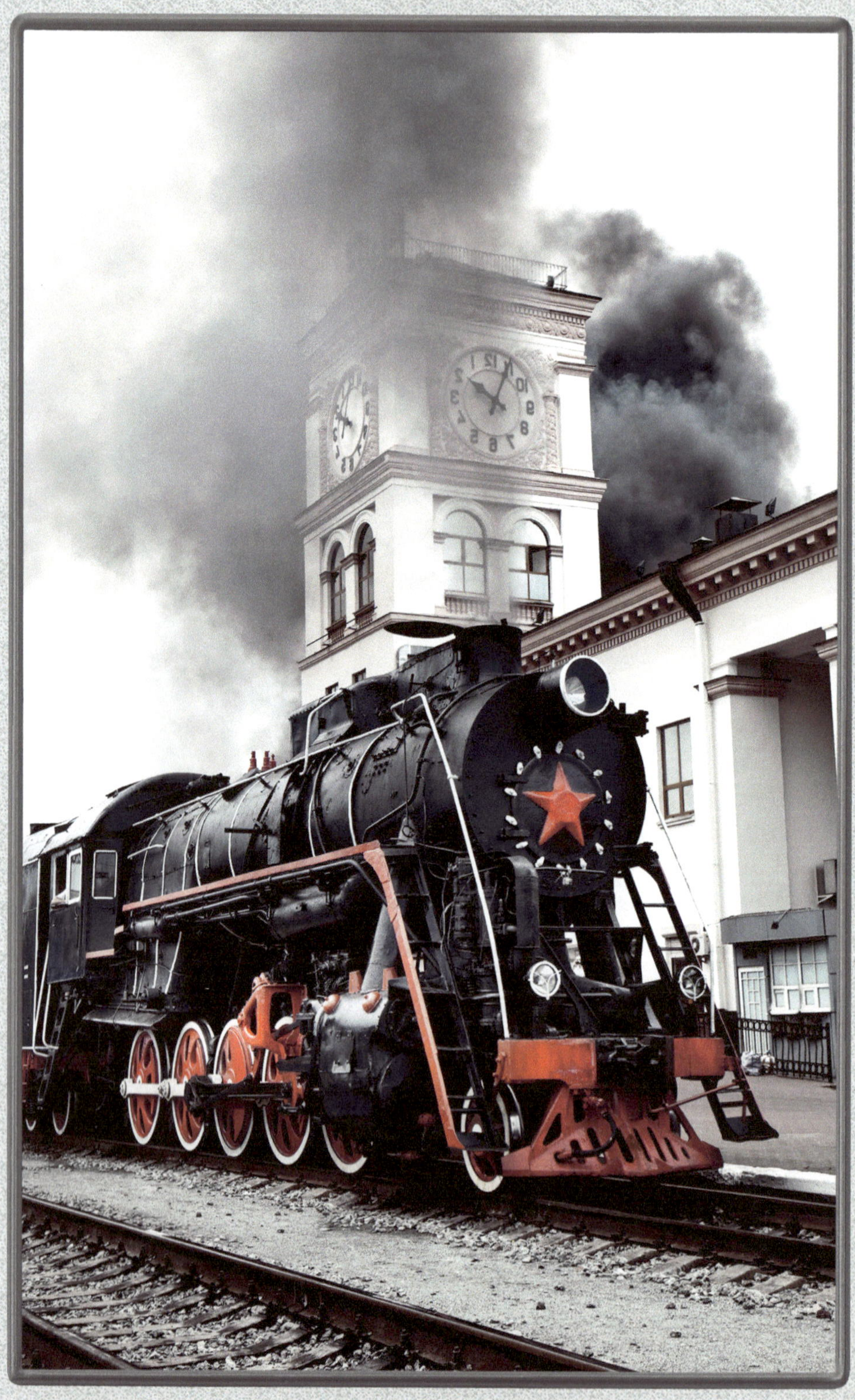

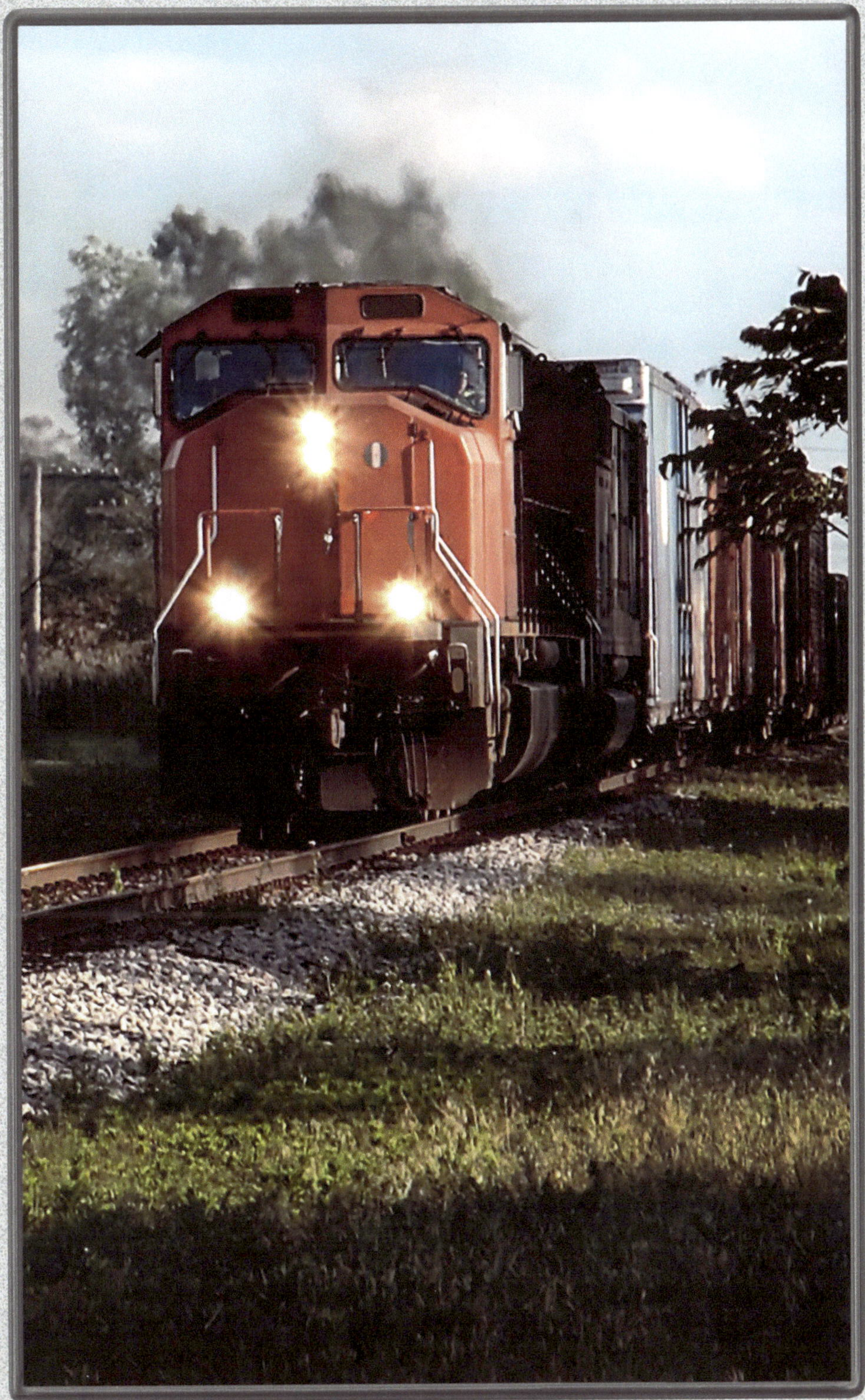

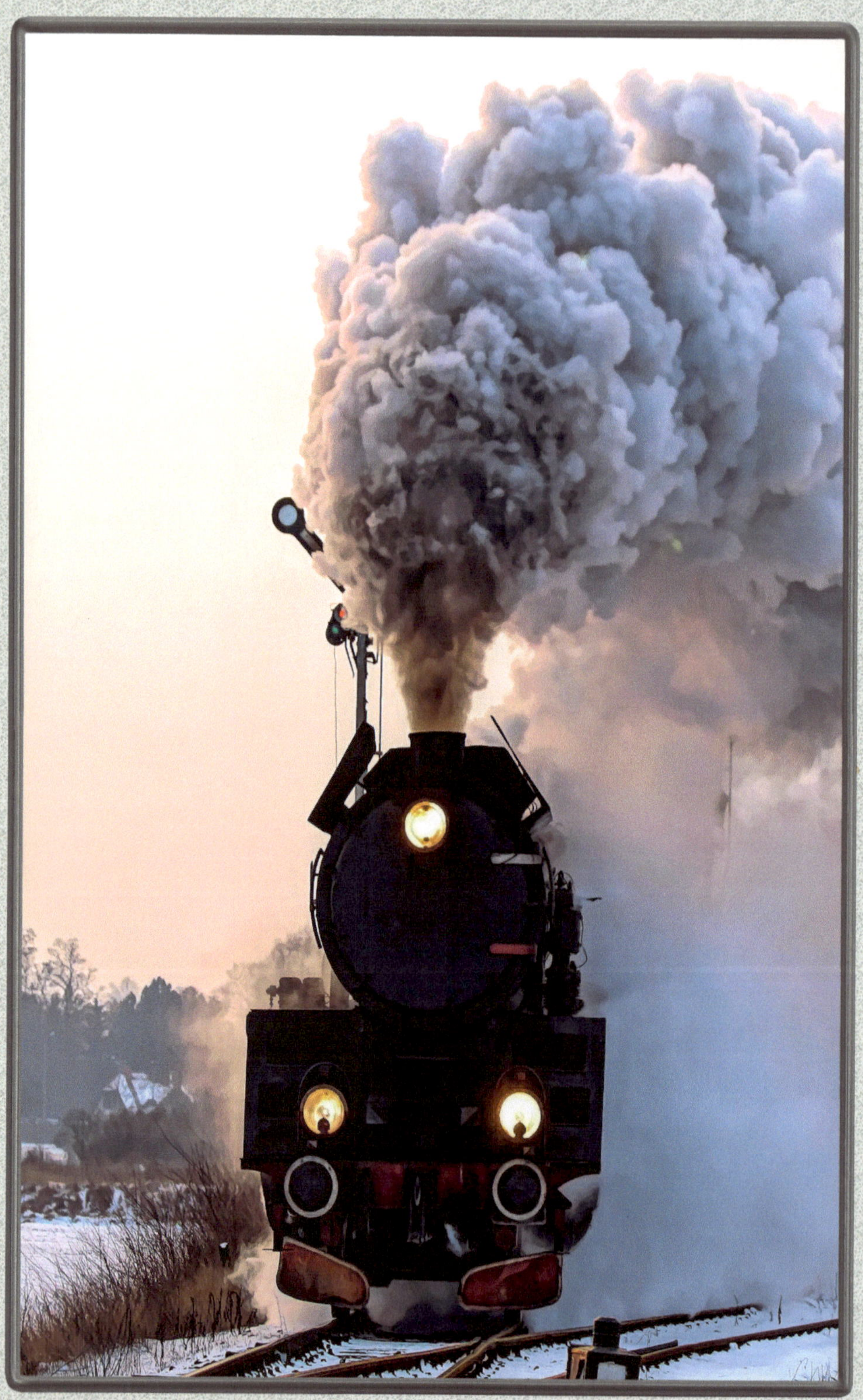

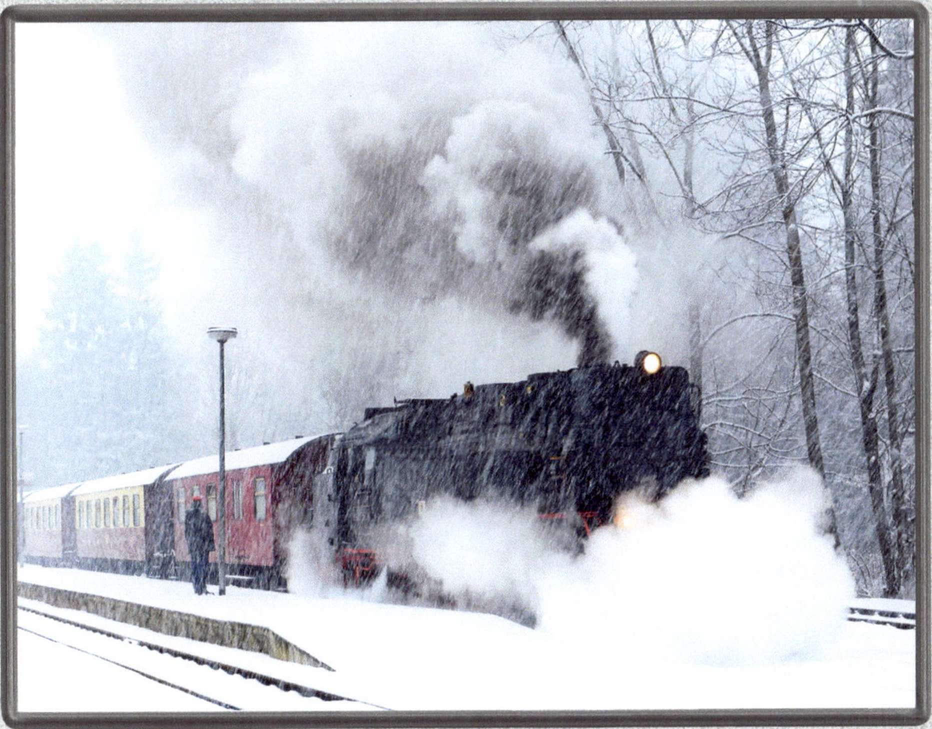

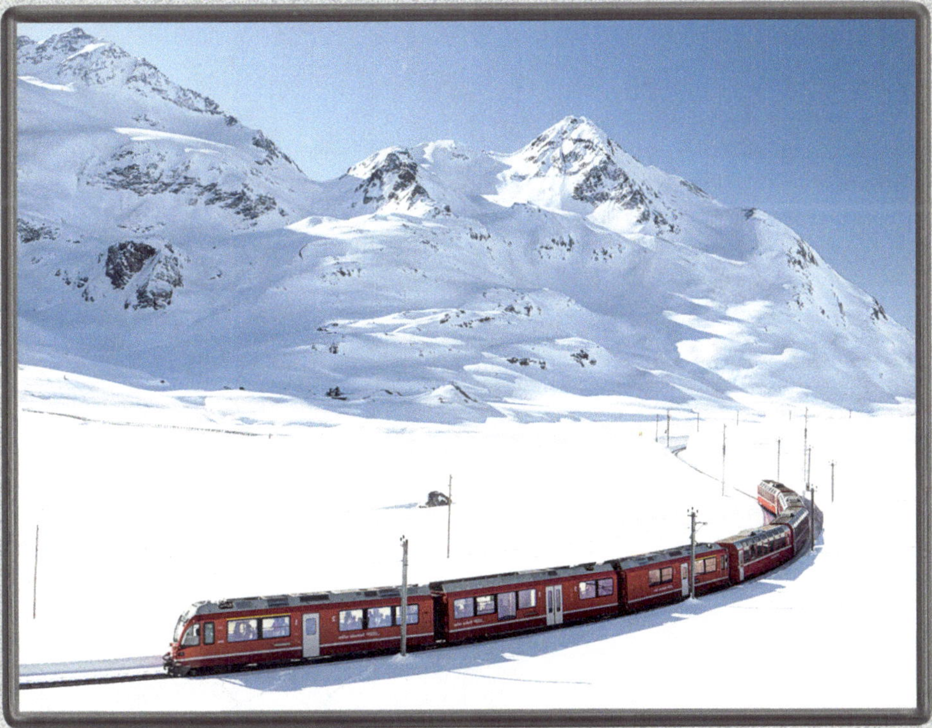

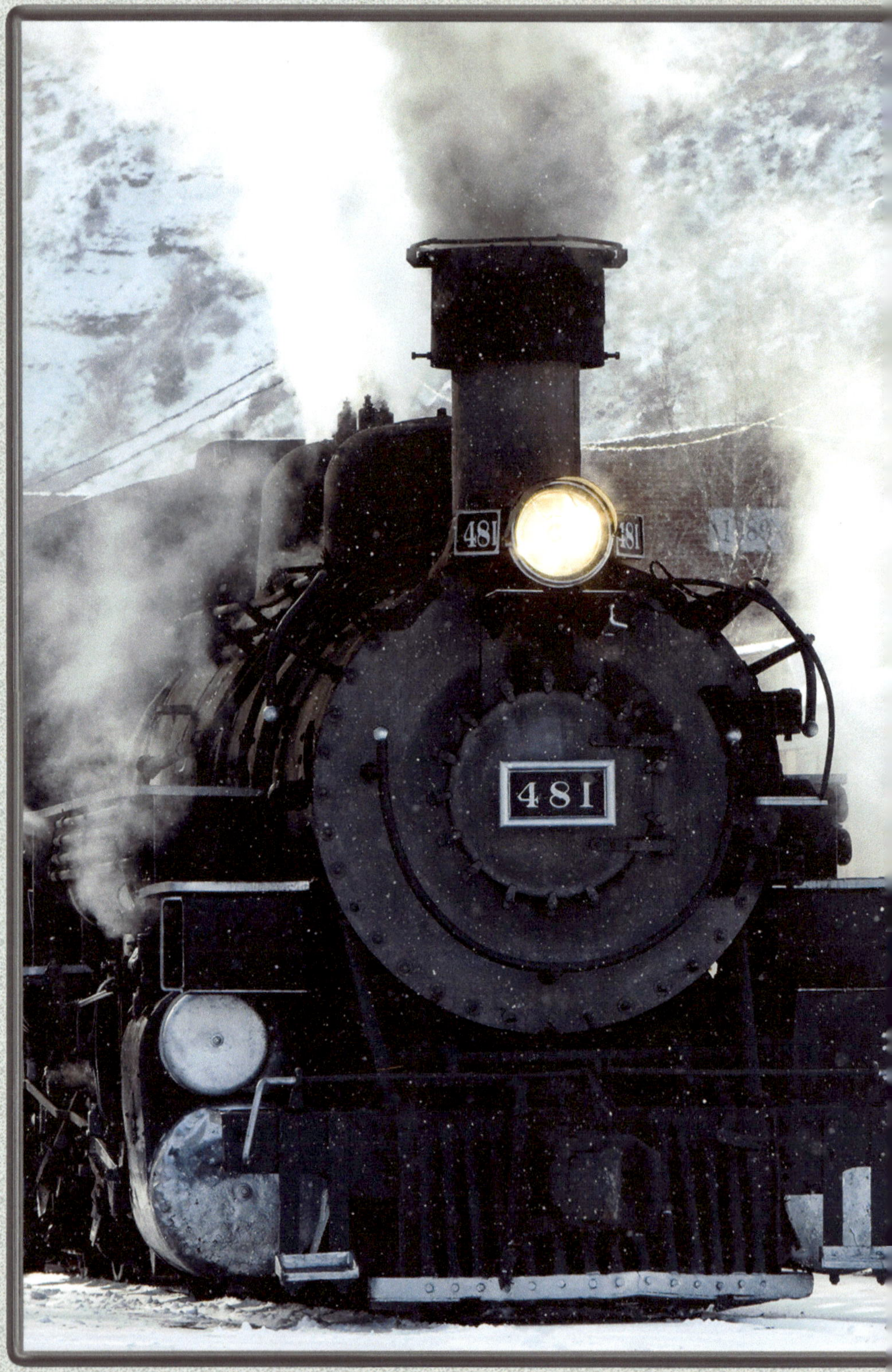
481
481
481

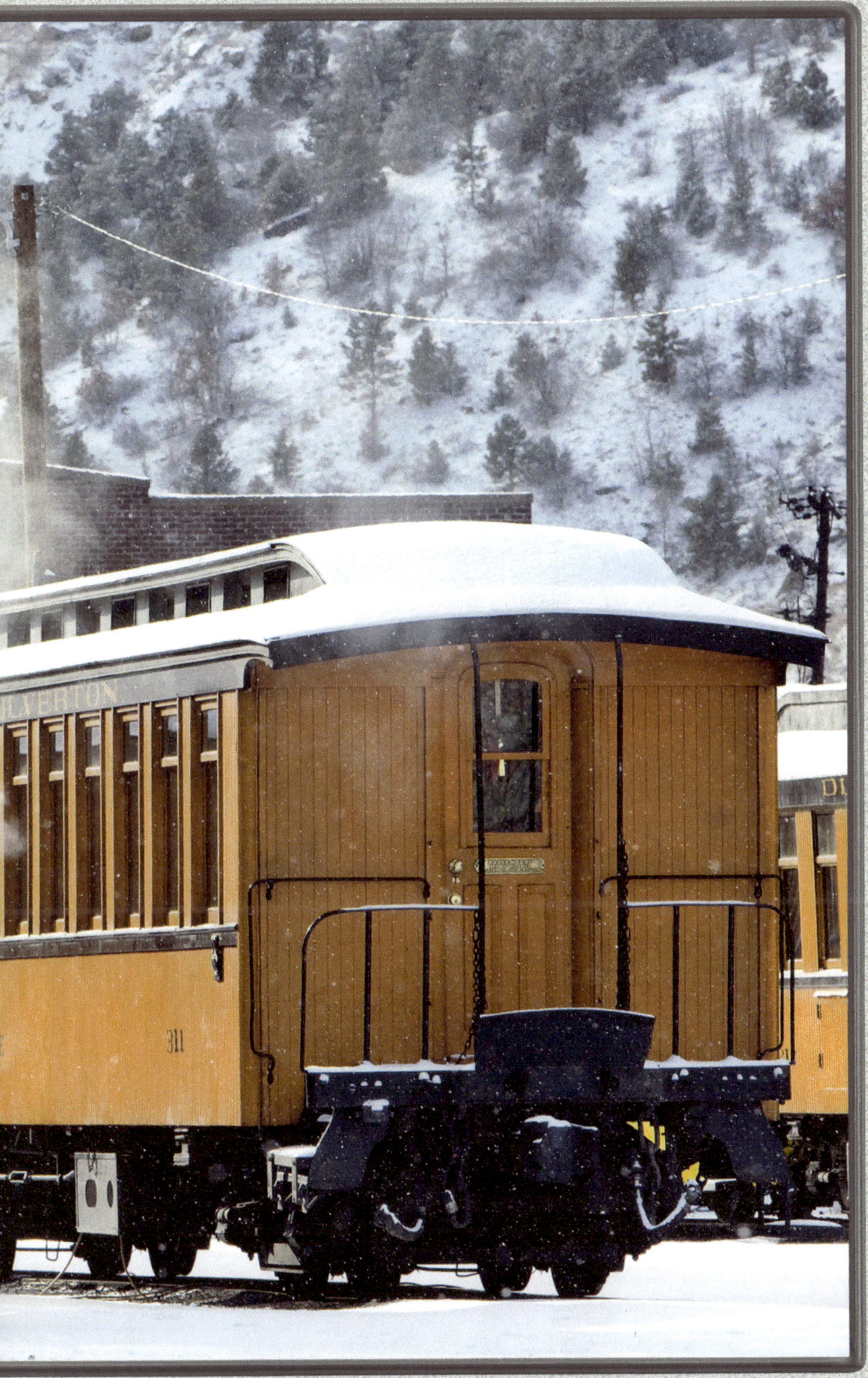

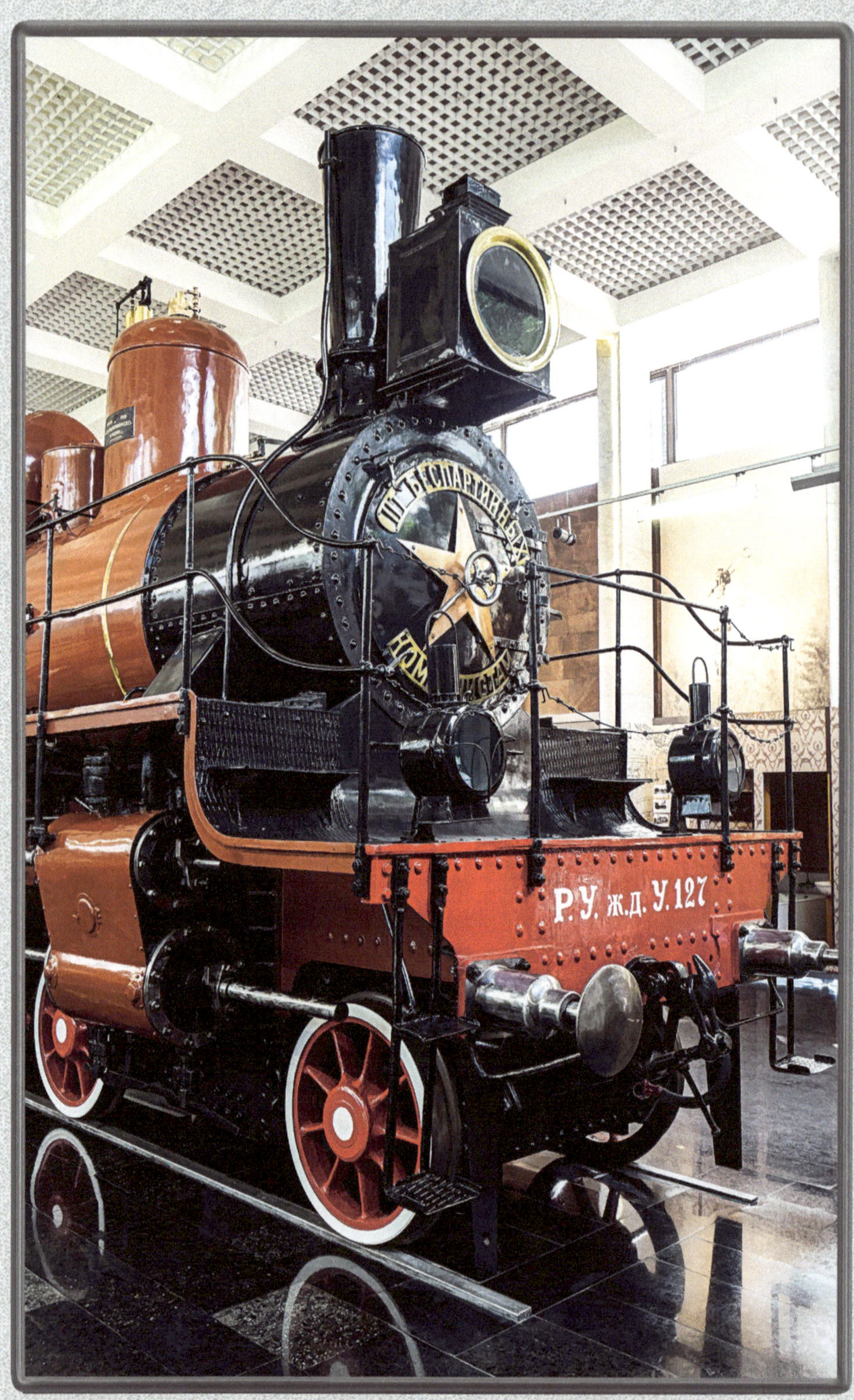
БЕСПАРТІЙНЫЙ
Р.У. ж.д. У. 127

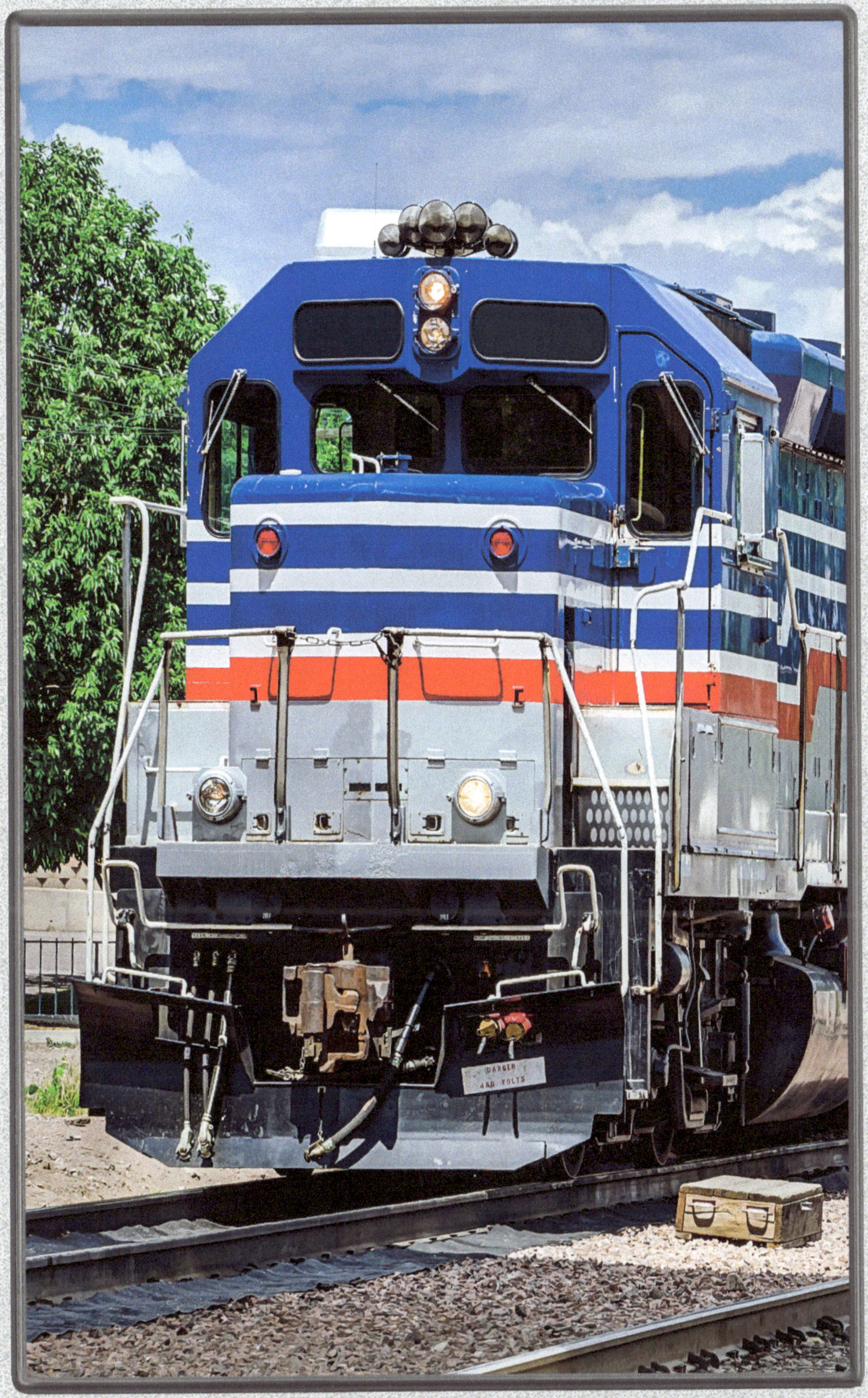

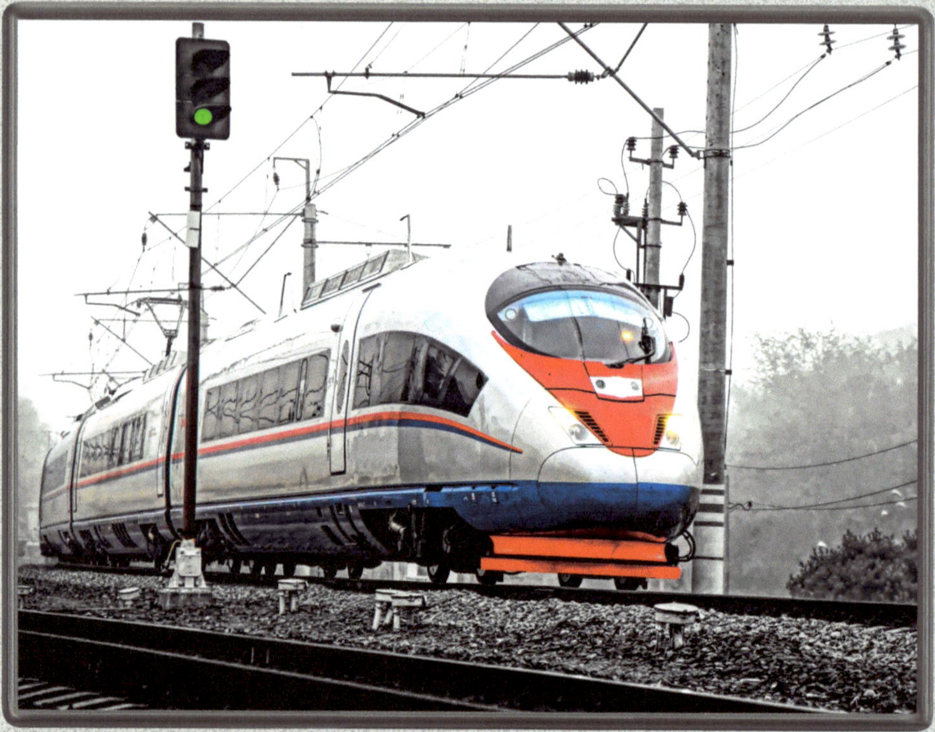

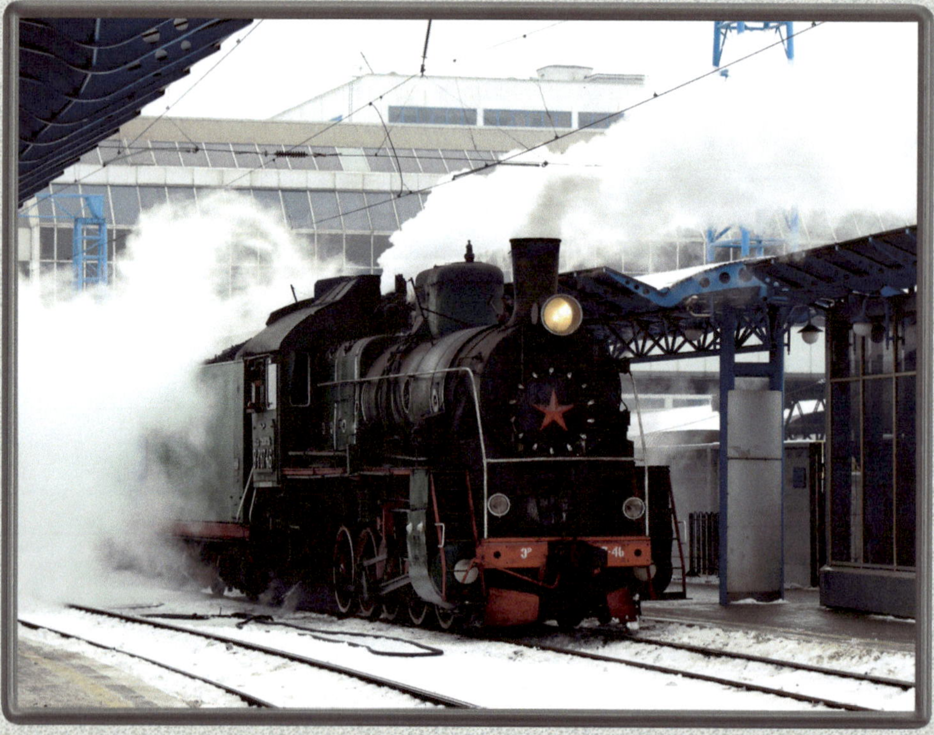

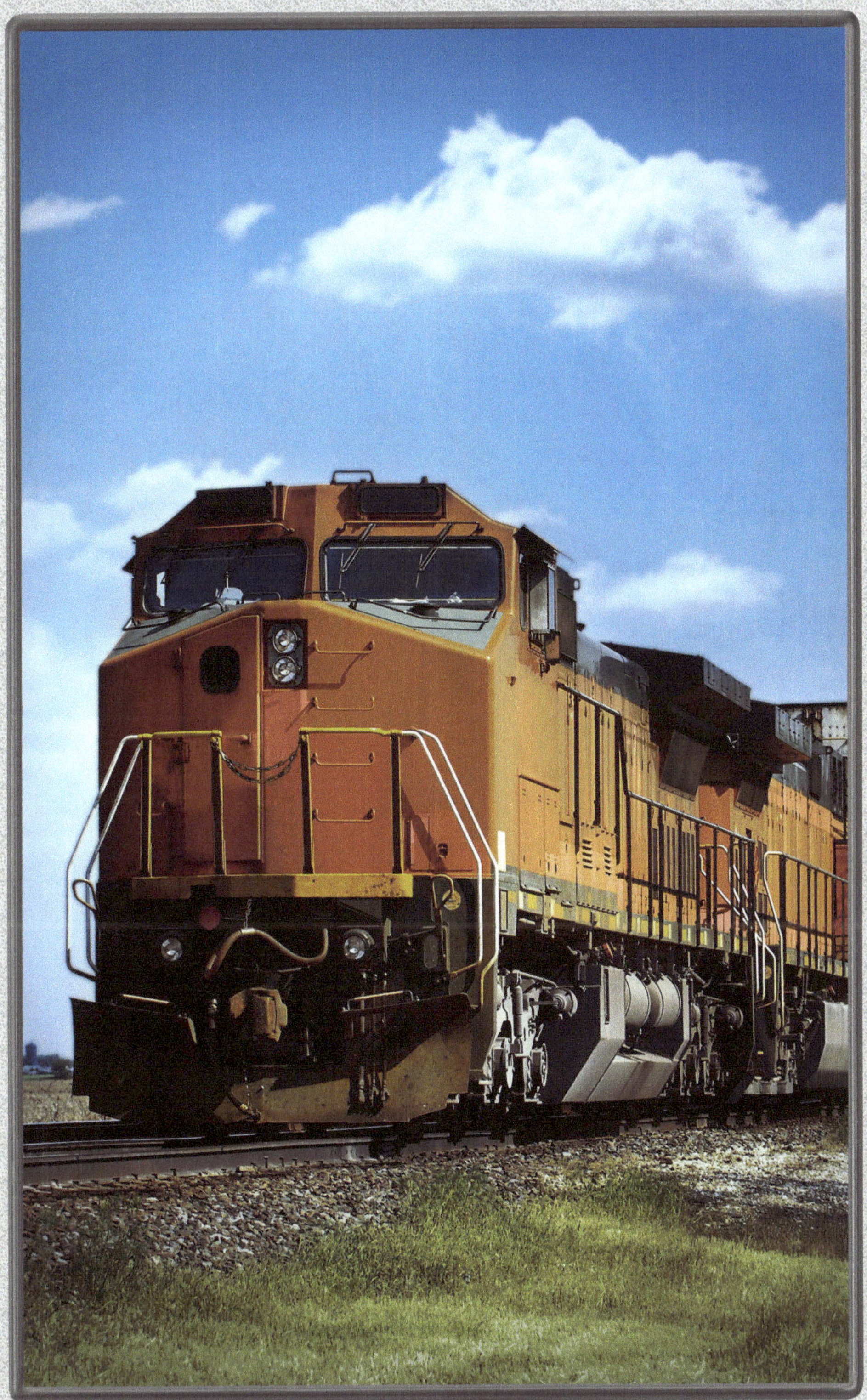

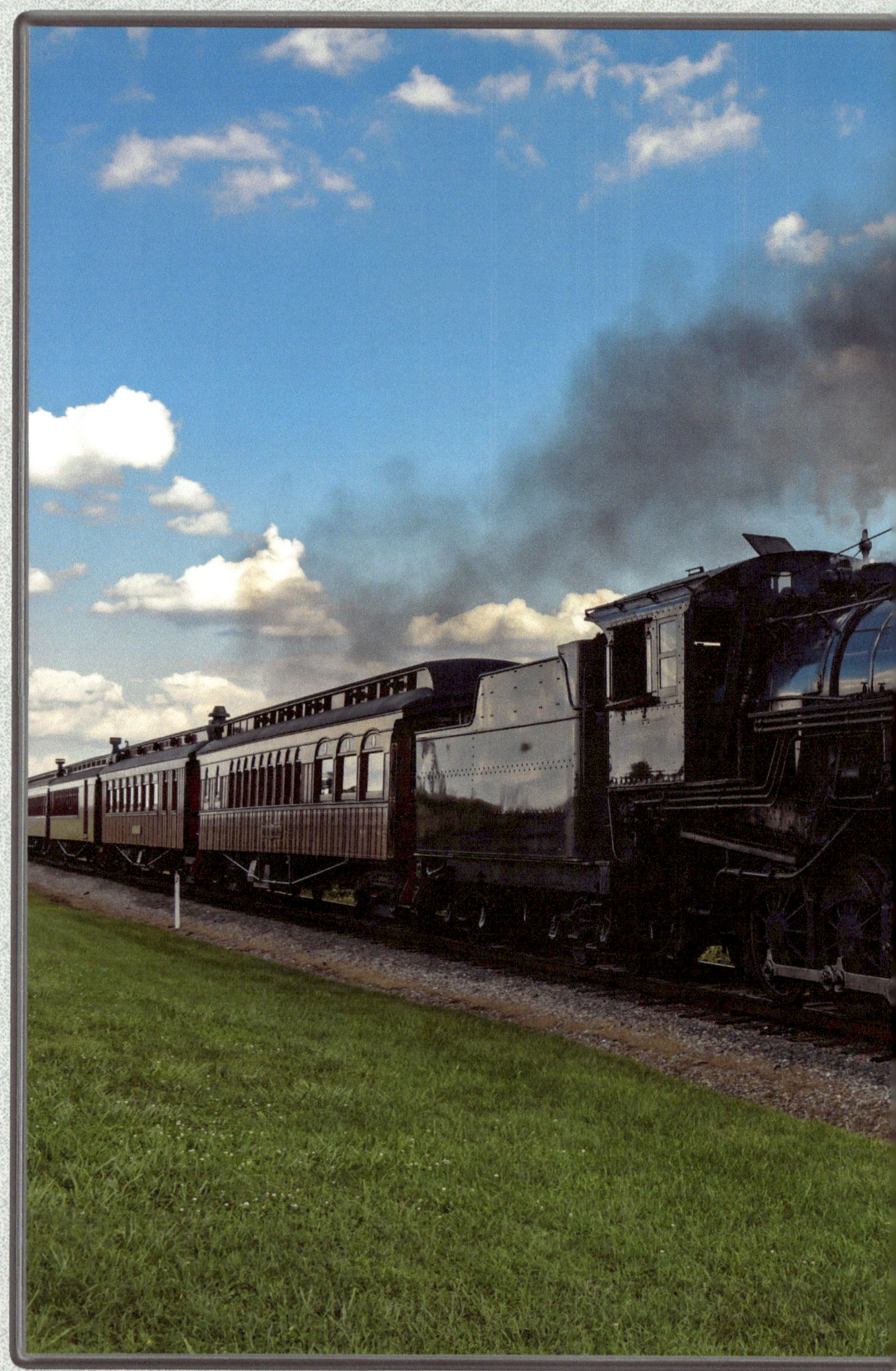

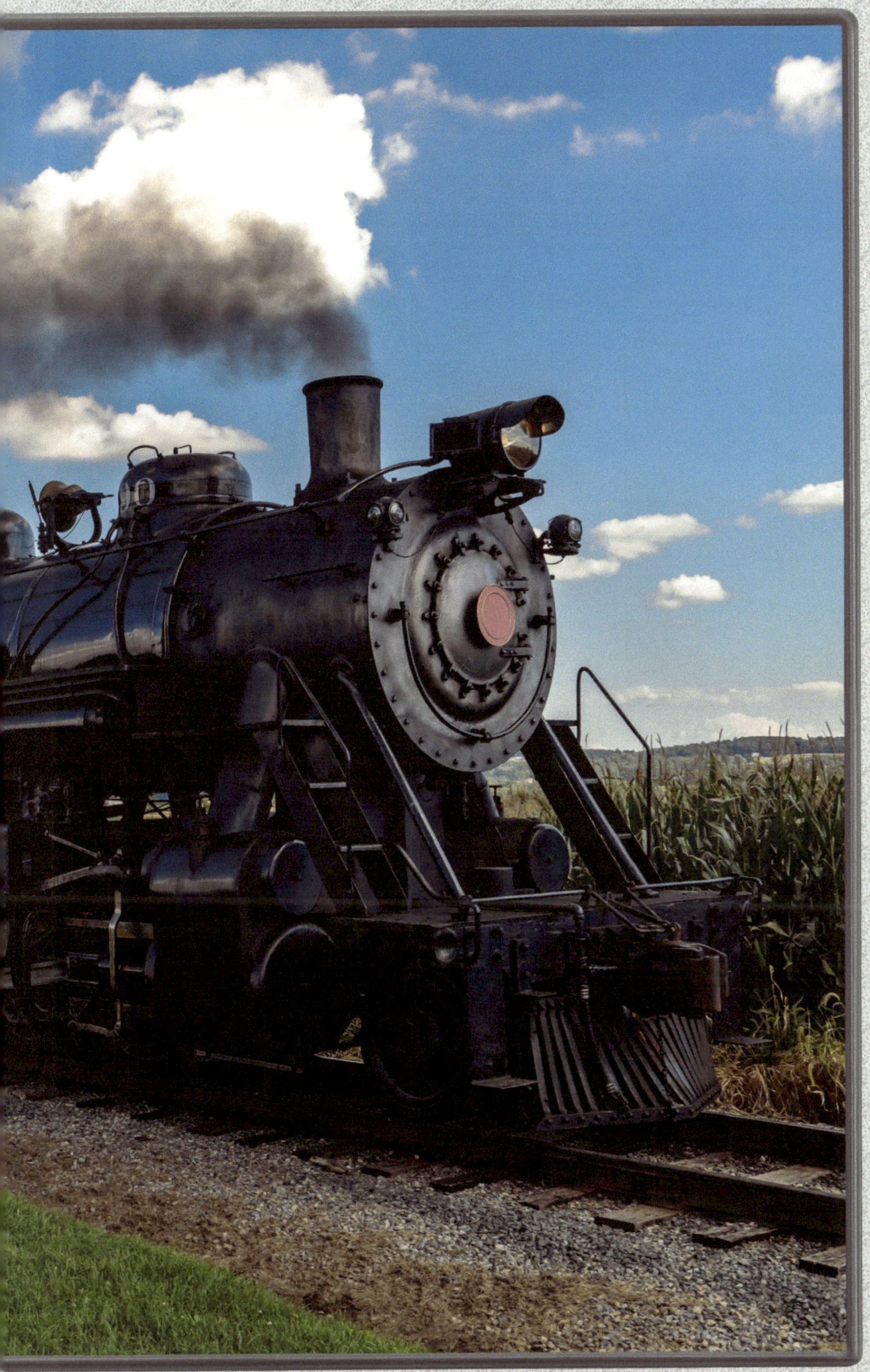

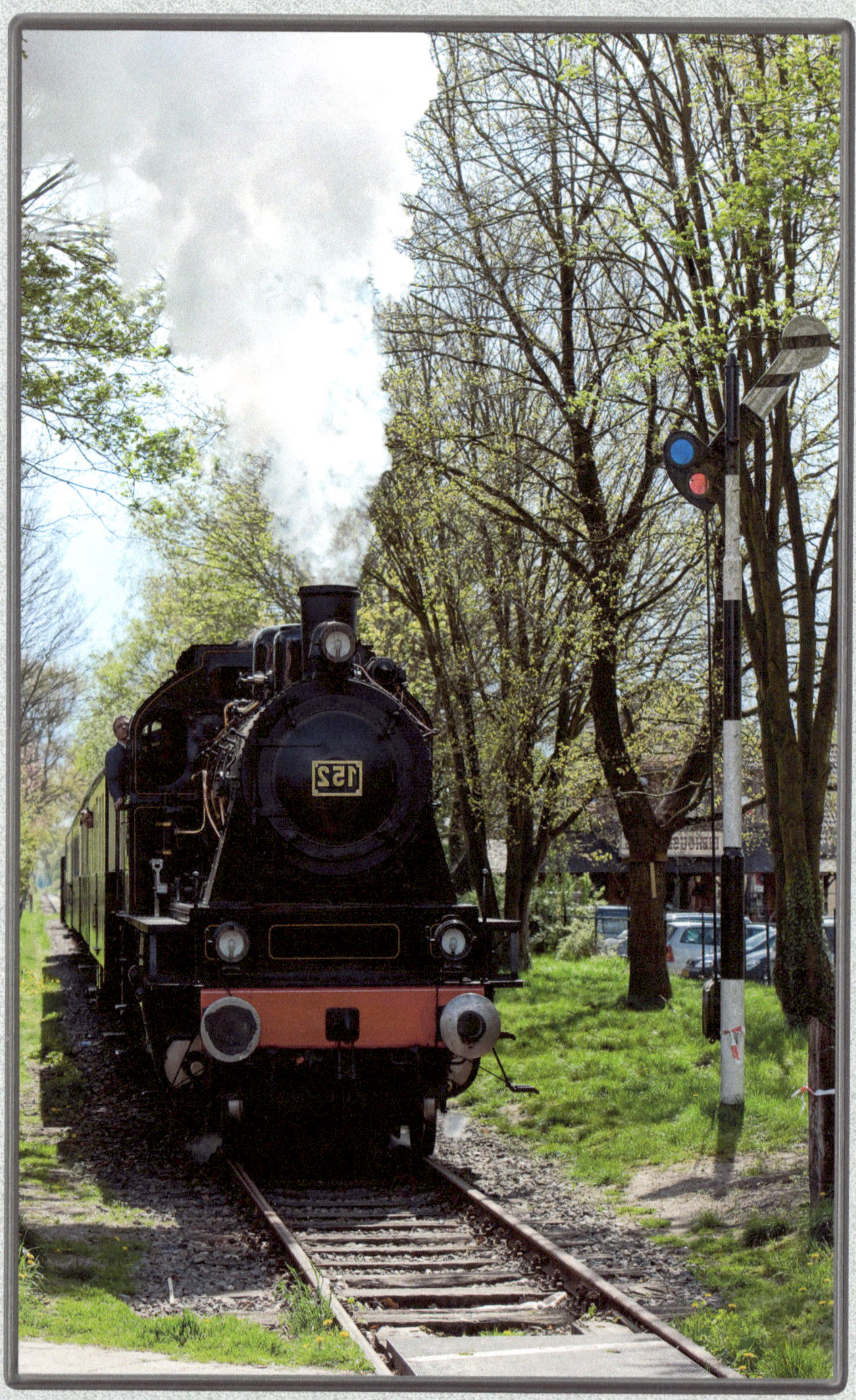

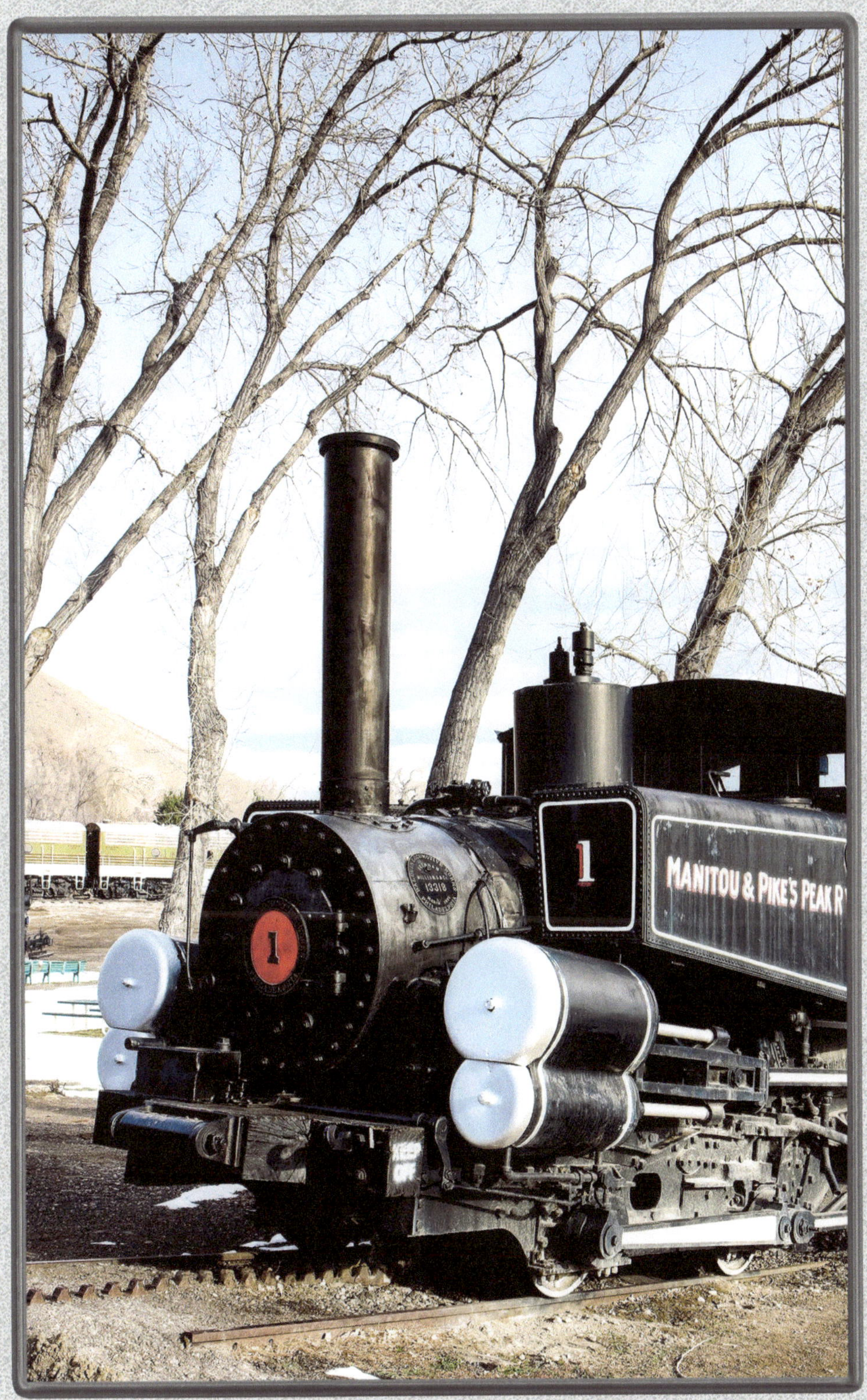
1
MANITOU & PIKE'S PEAK R'

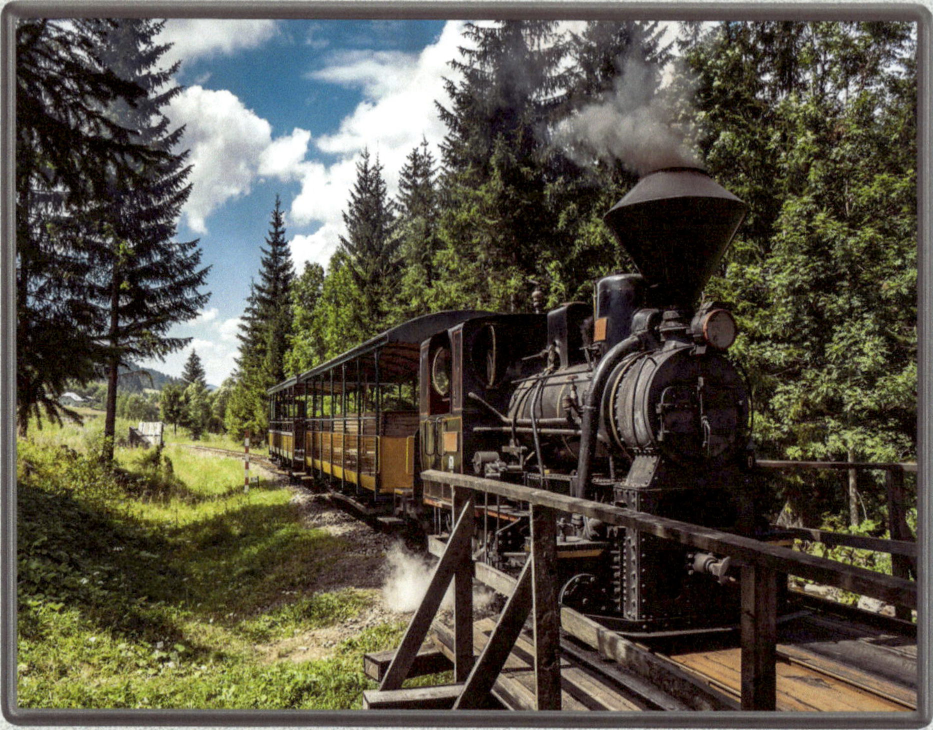

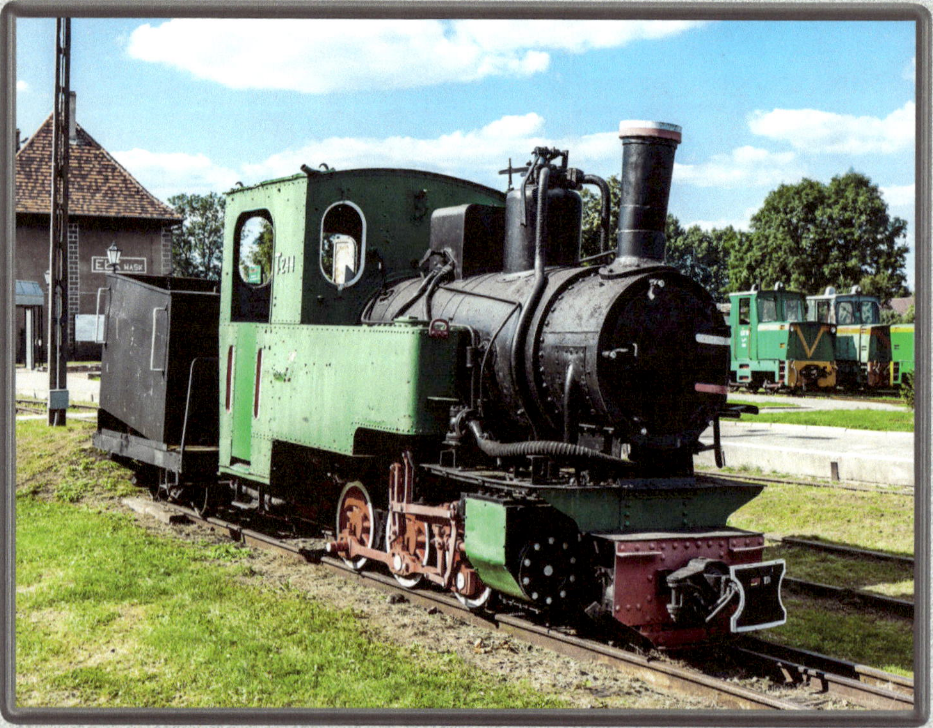

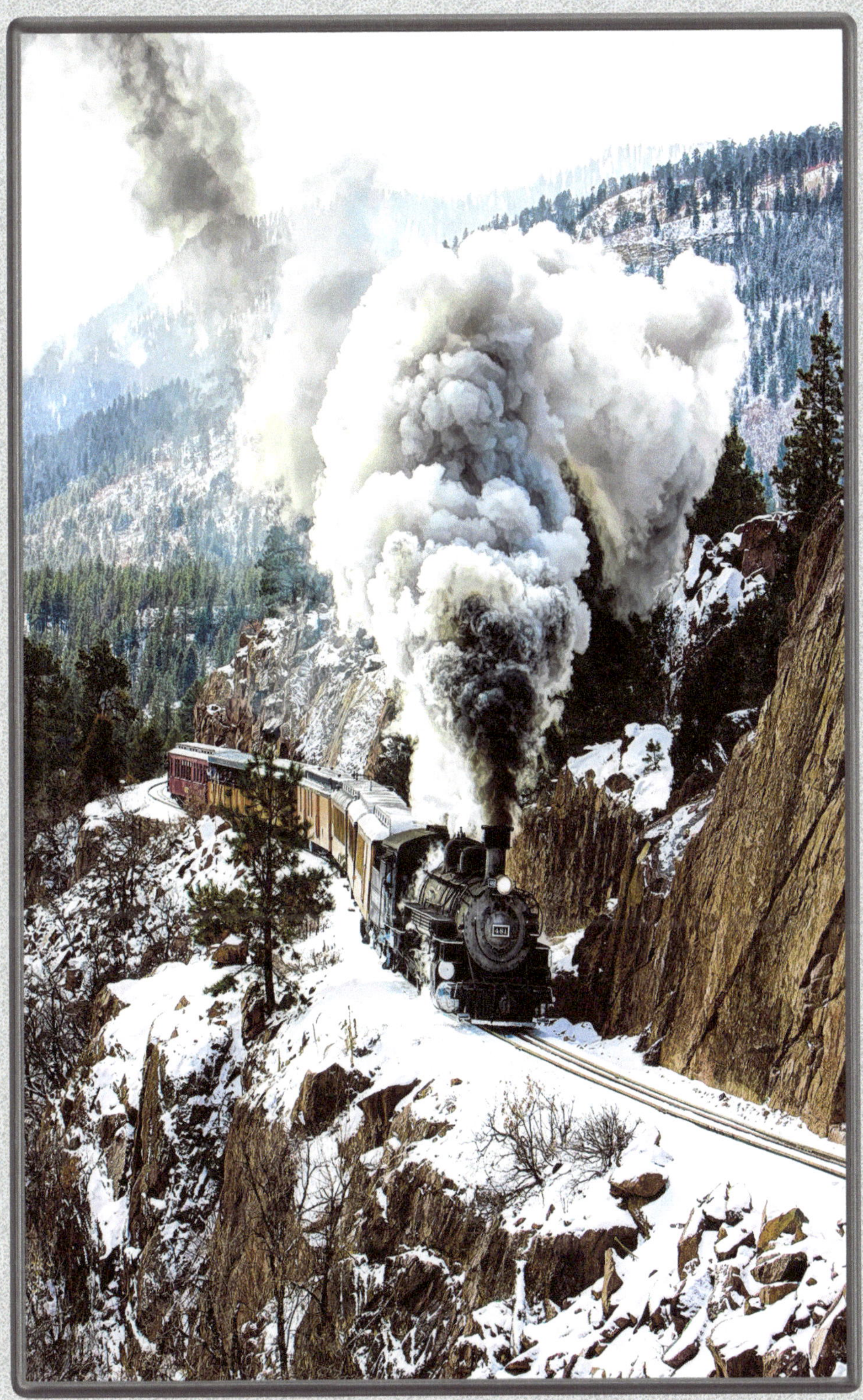

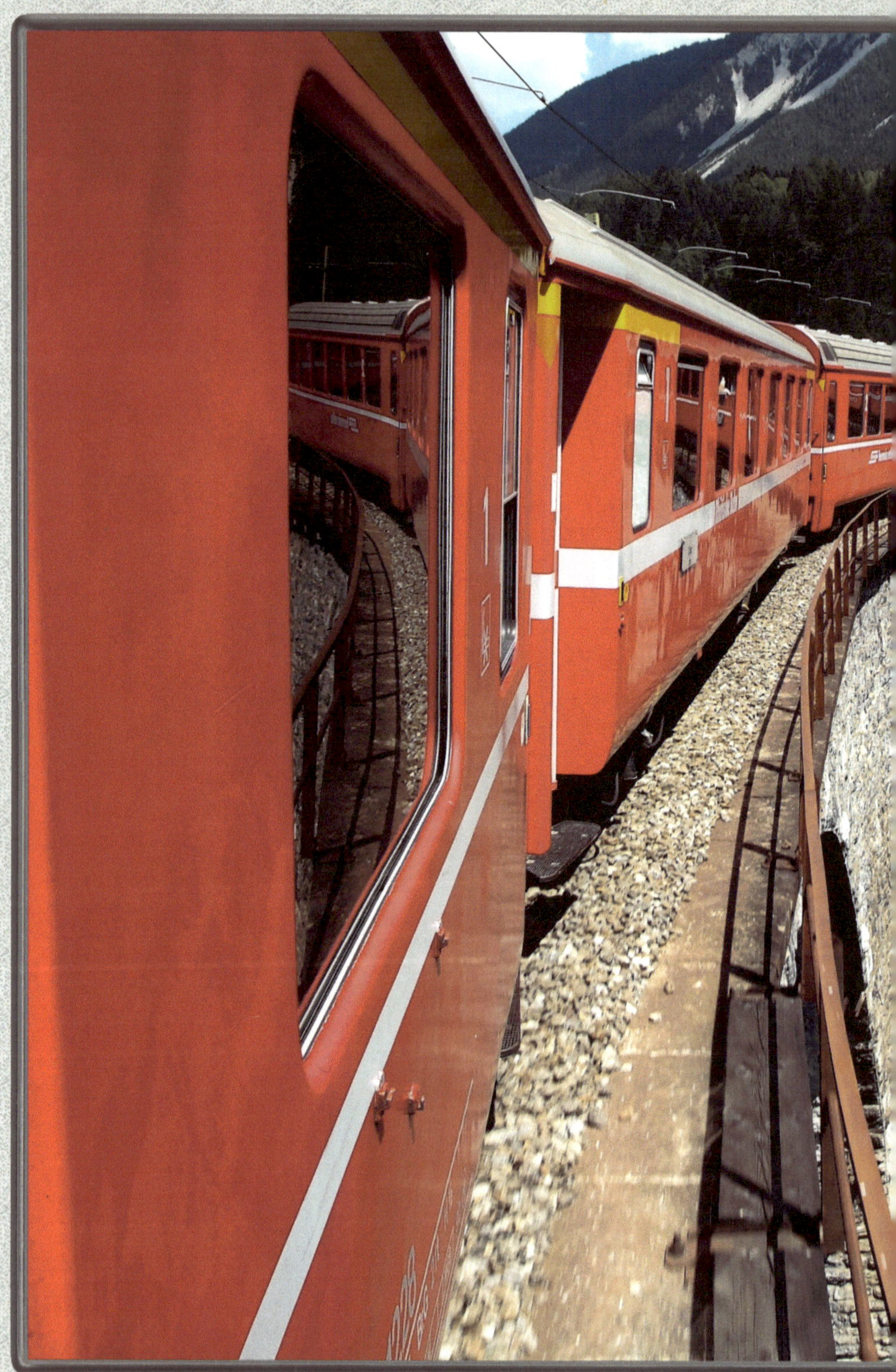

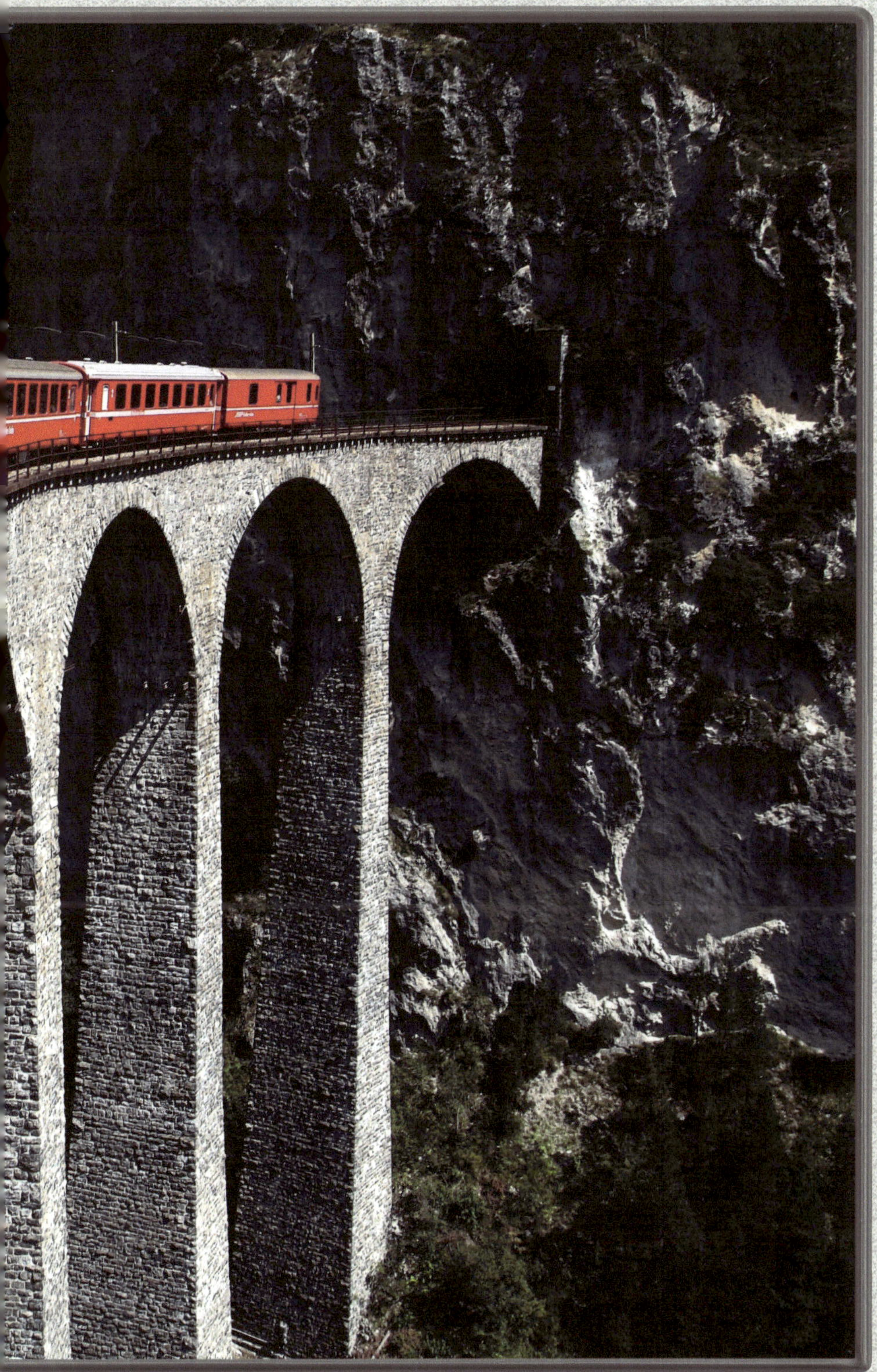

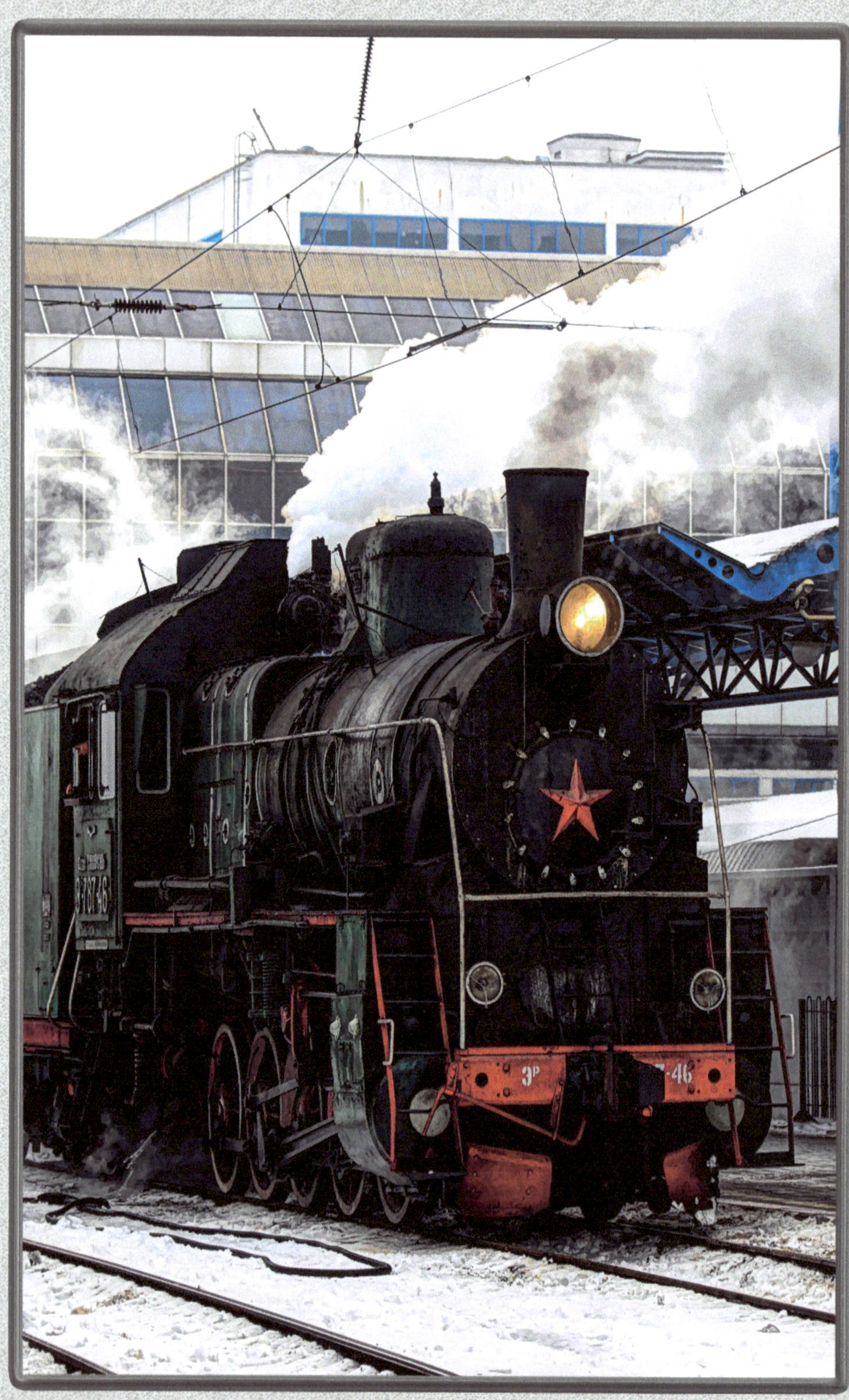

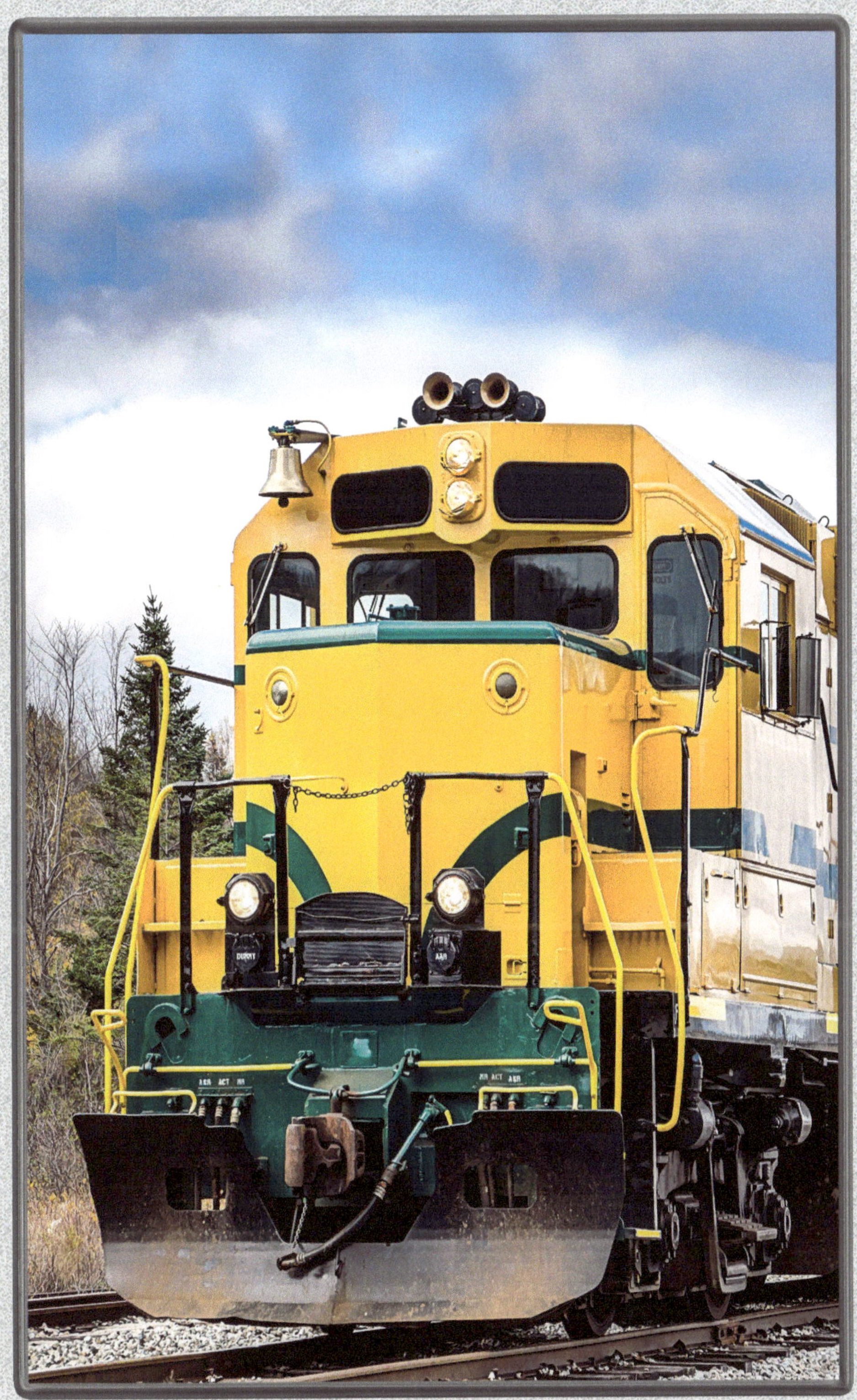

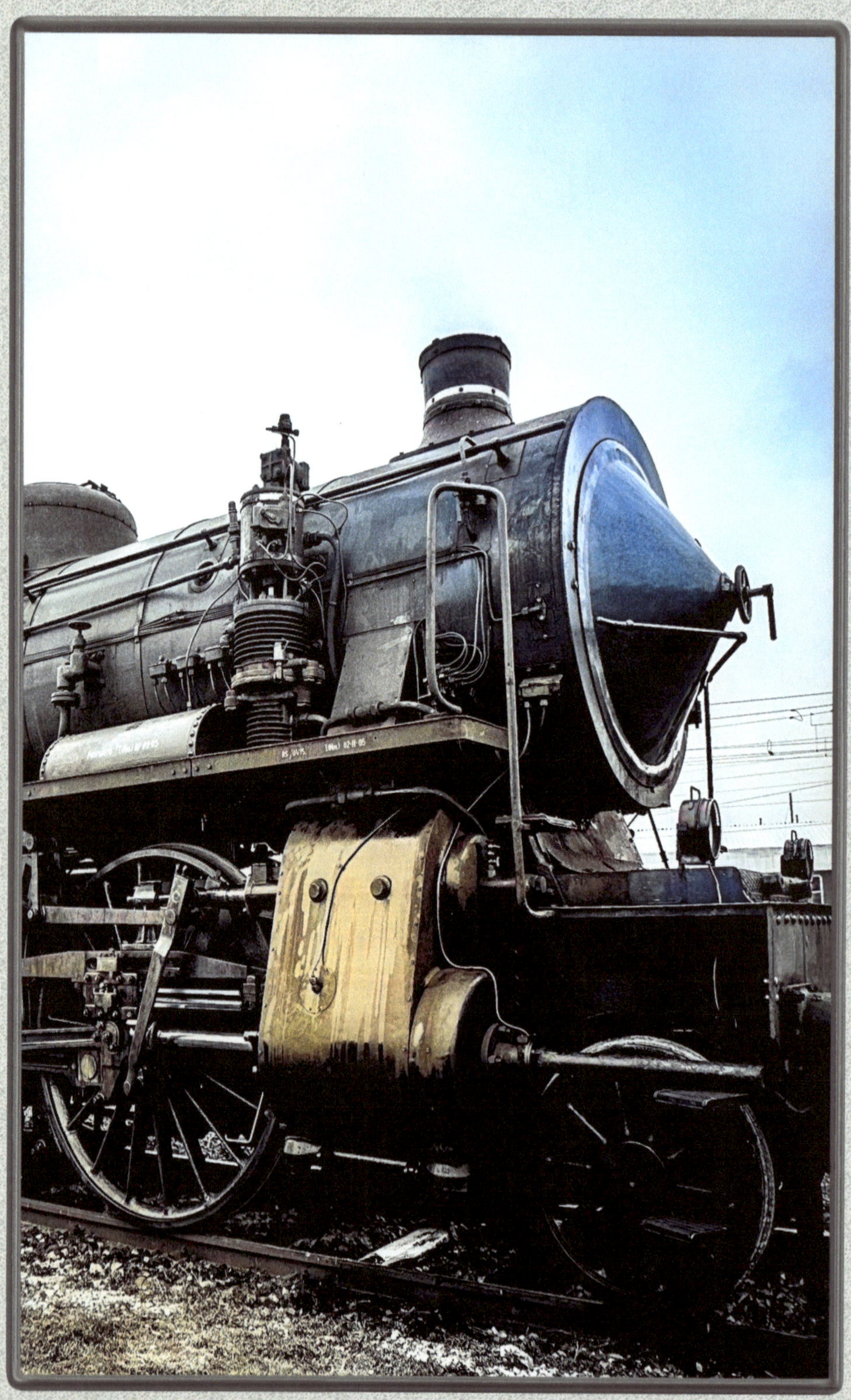

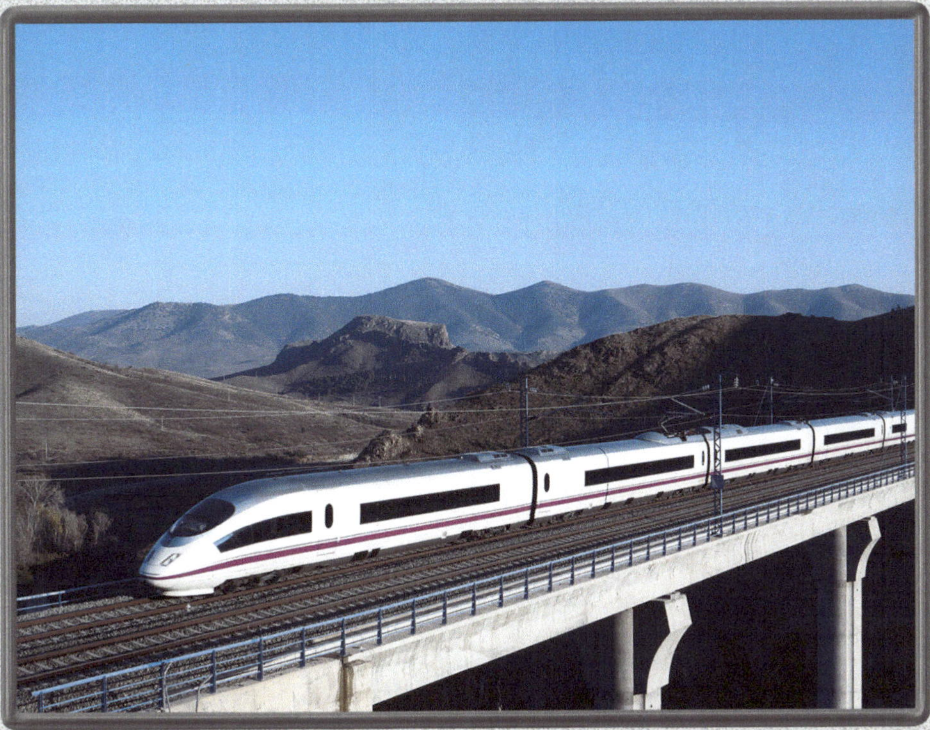

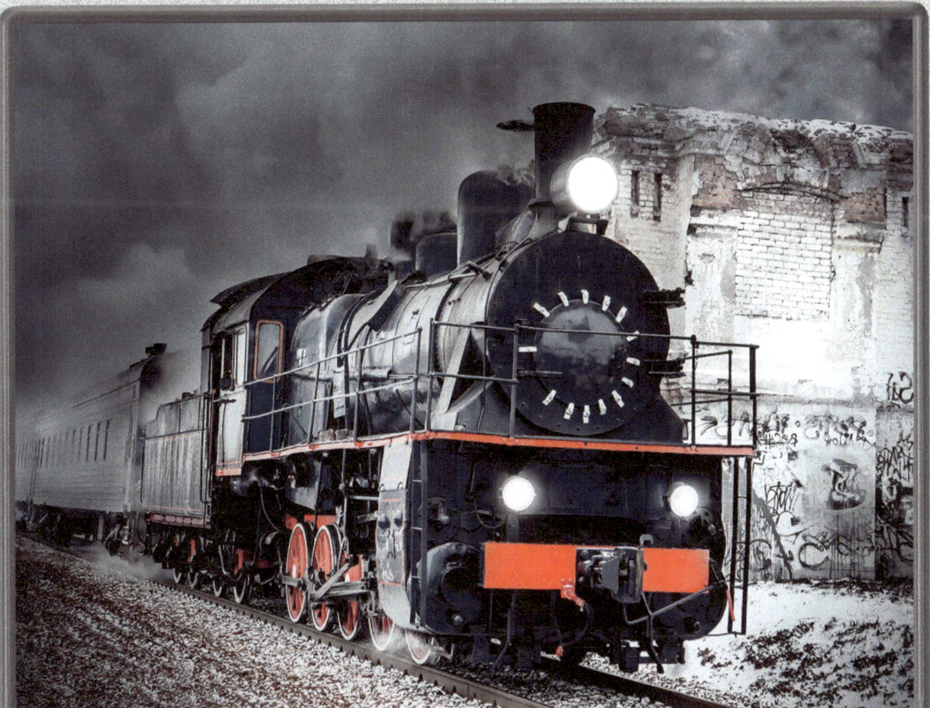

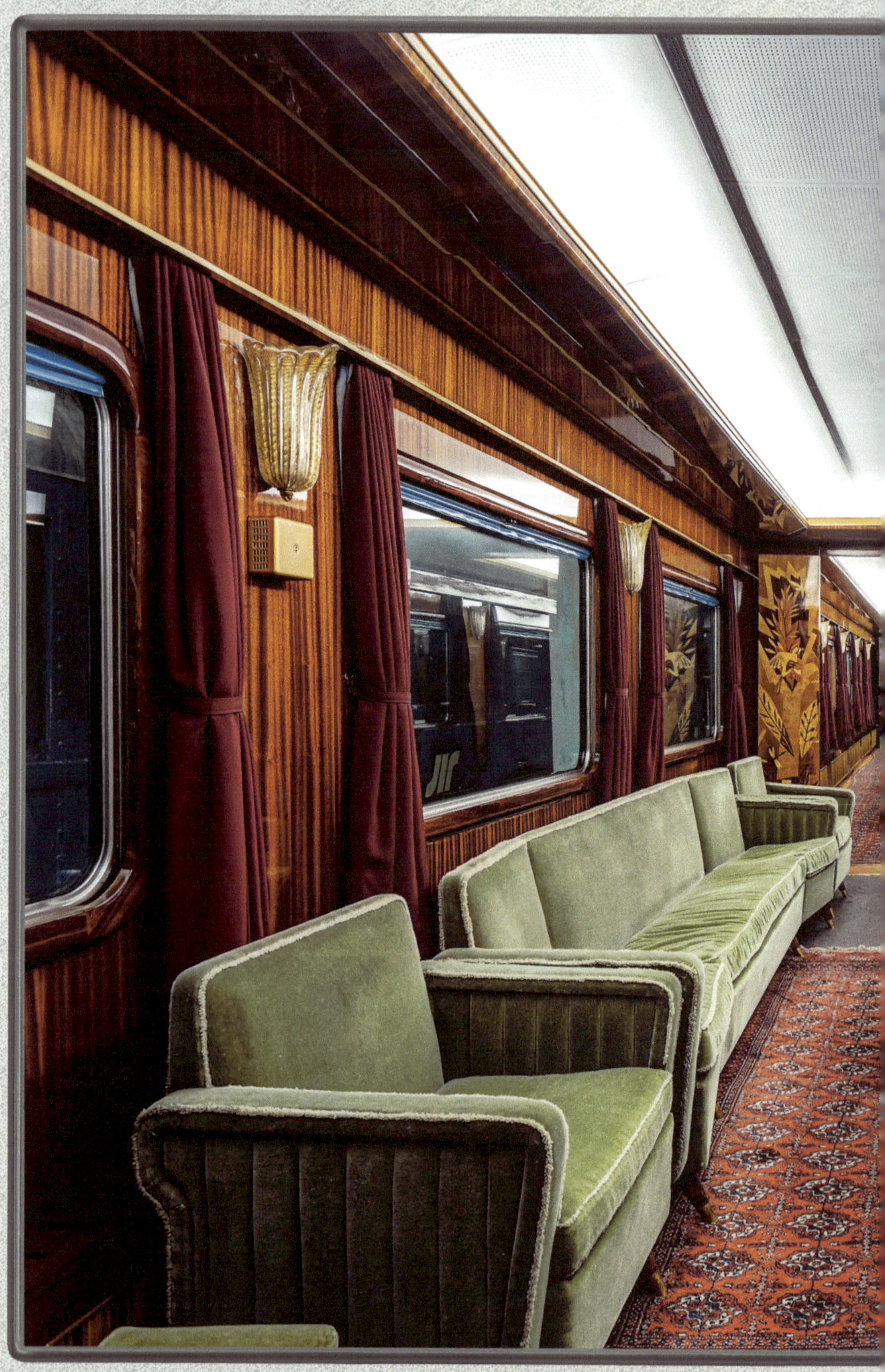

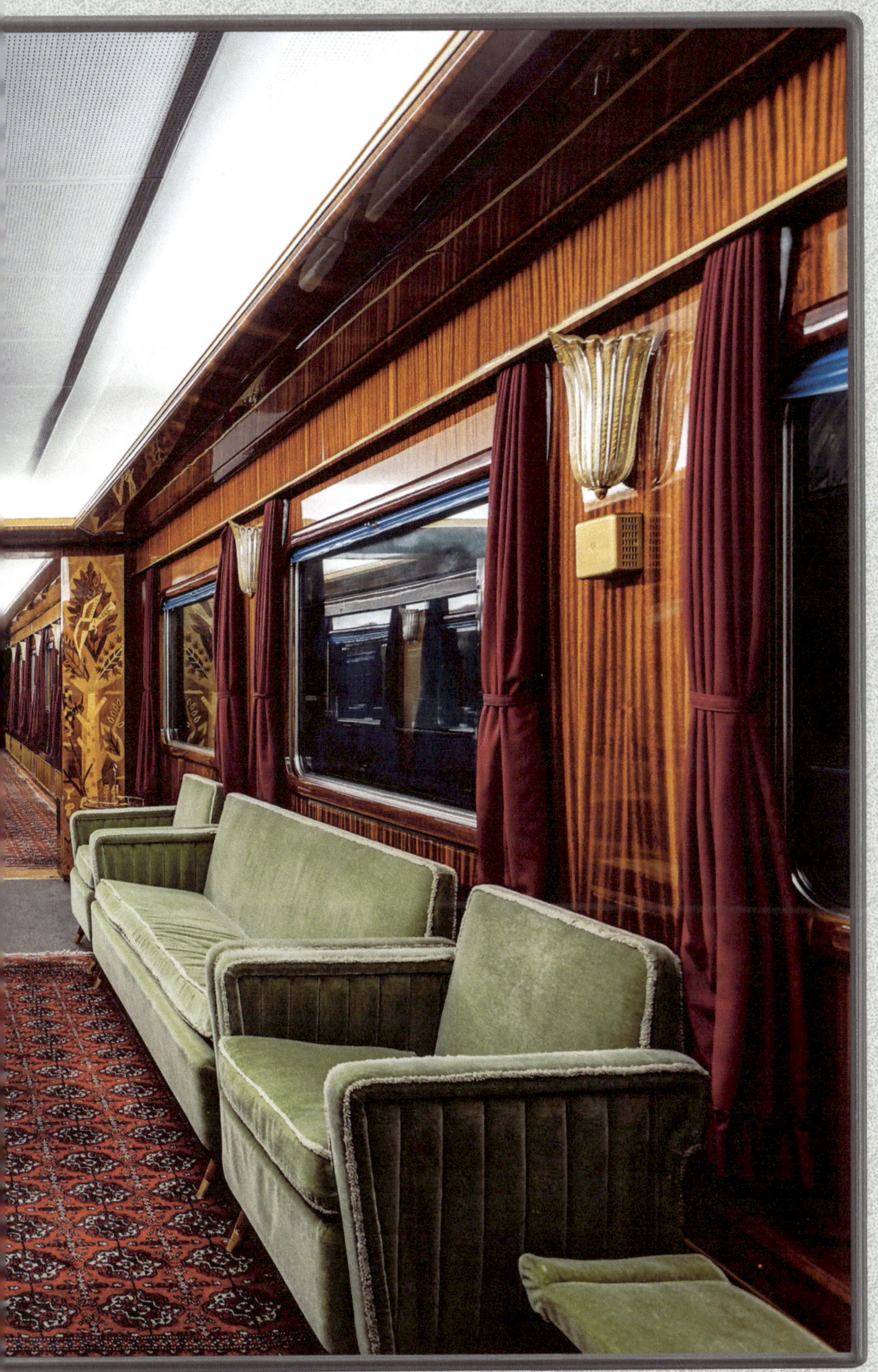

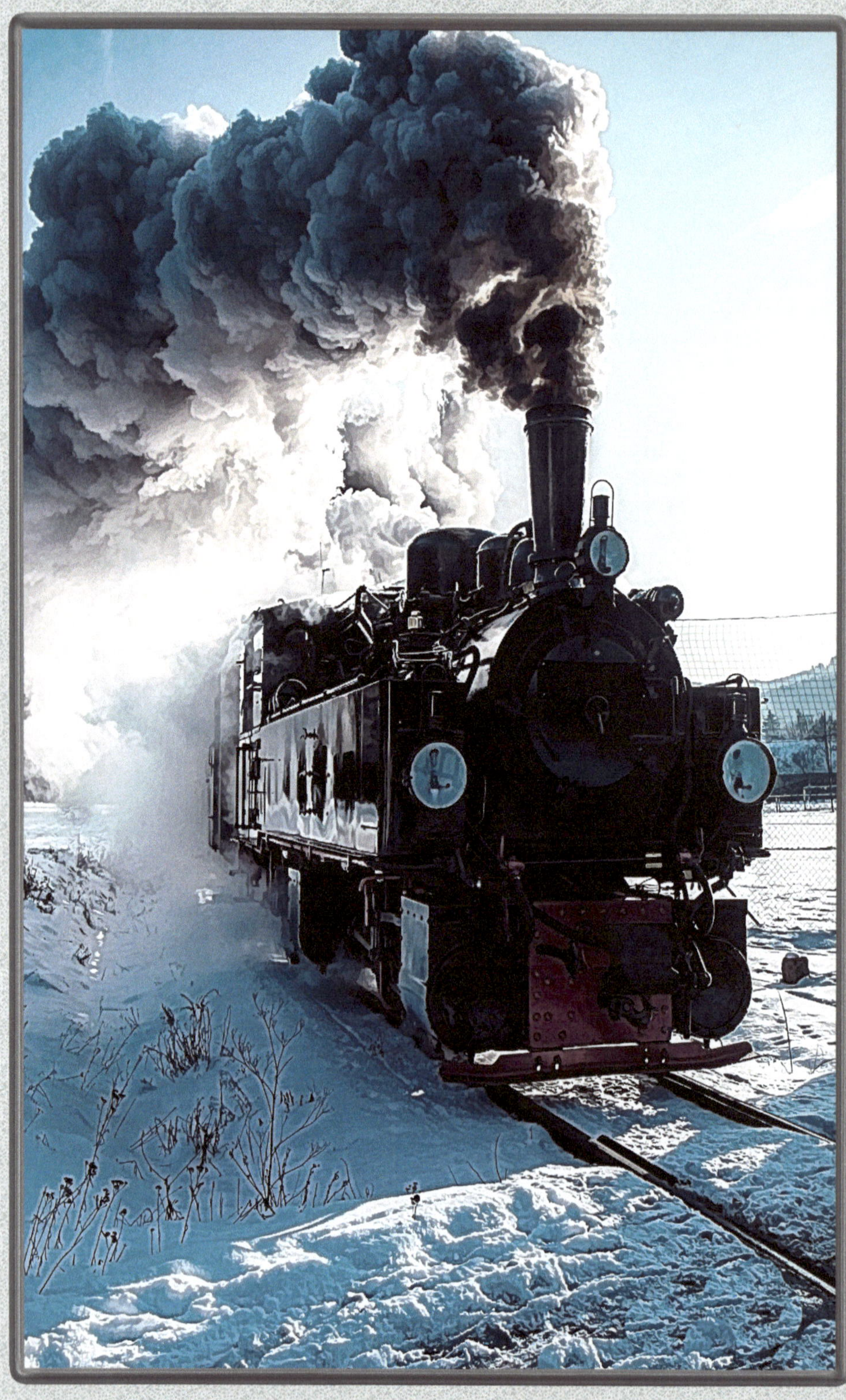

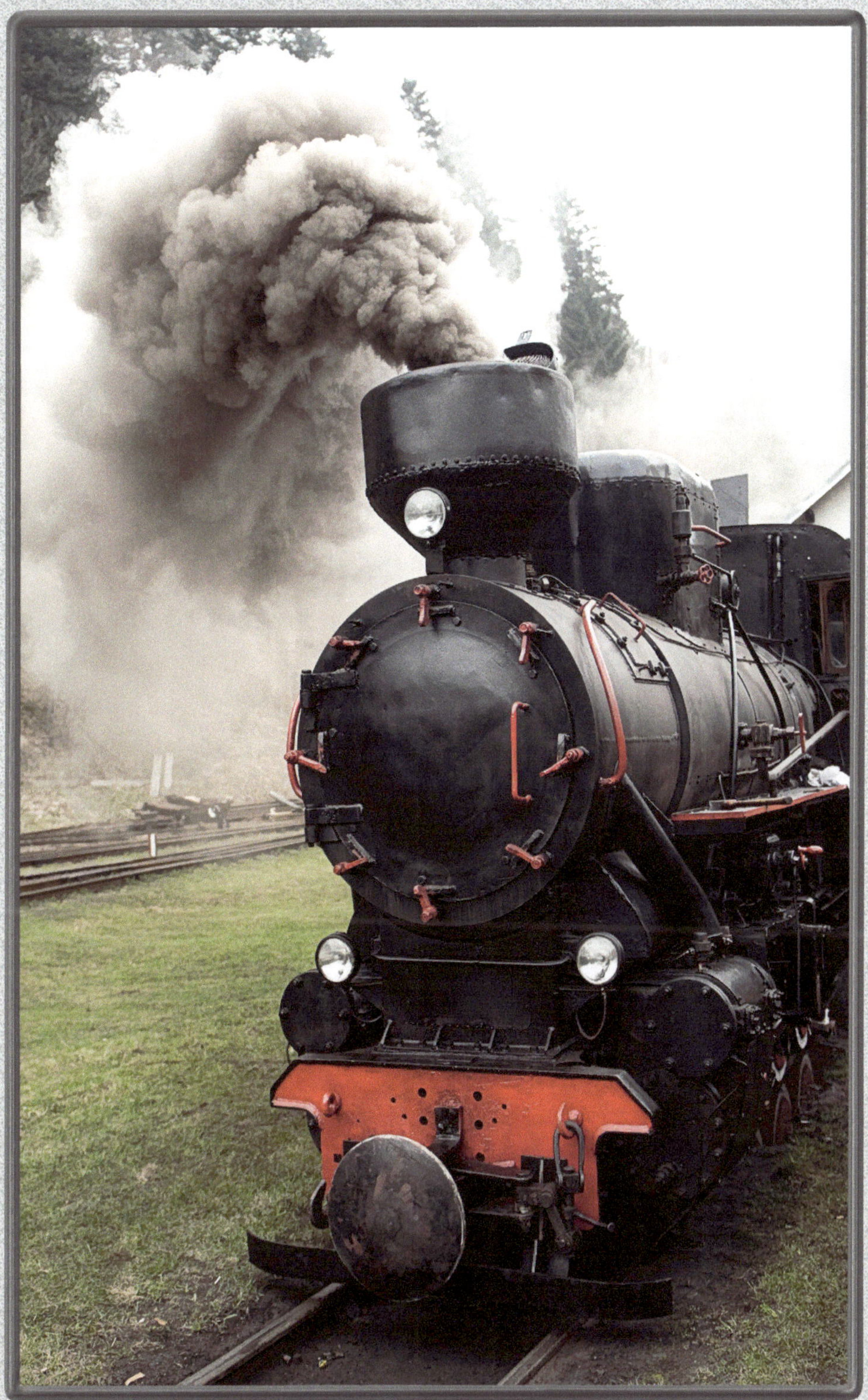

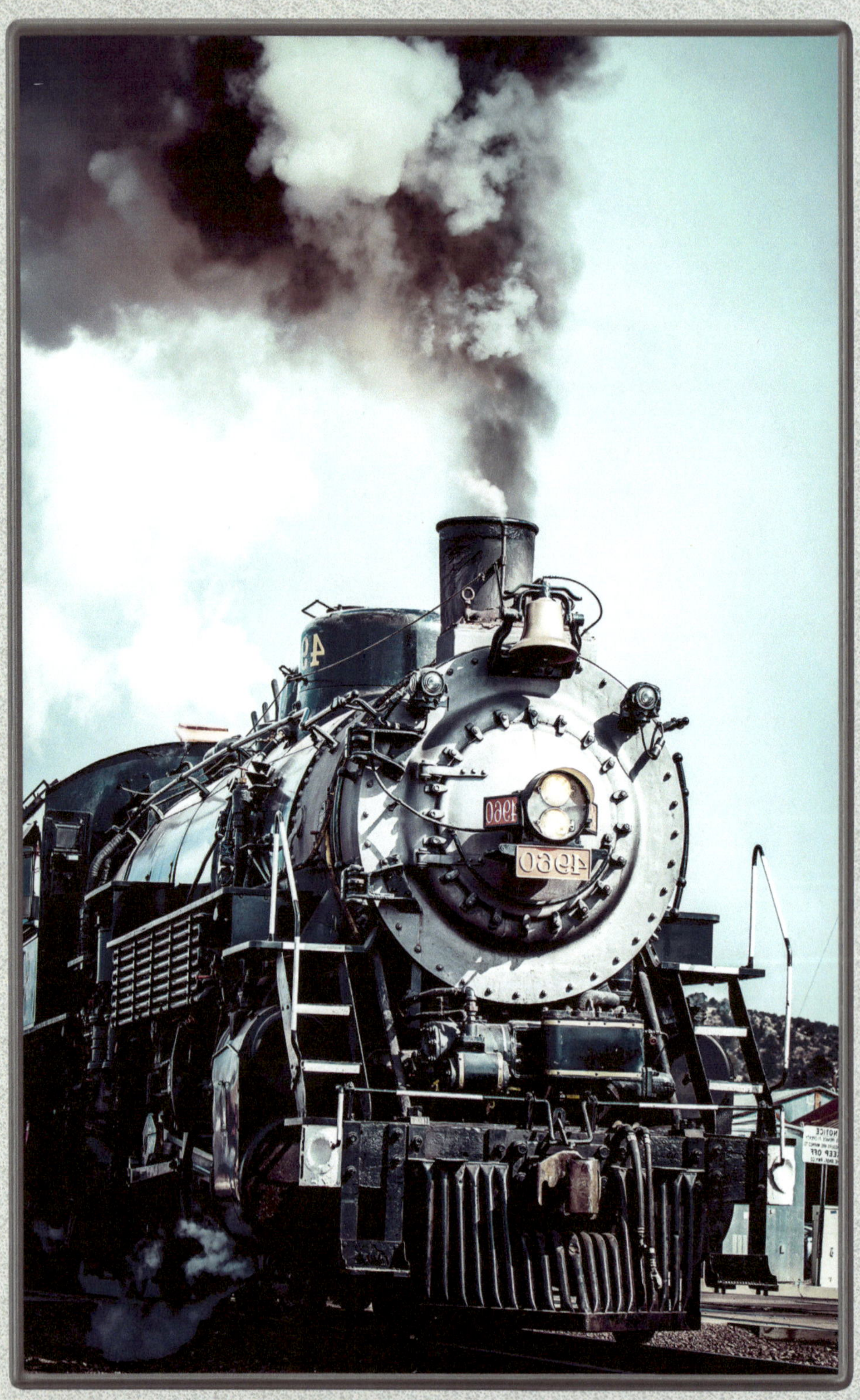
4960
NOTICE
KEEP OFF

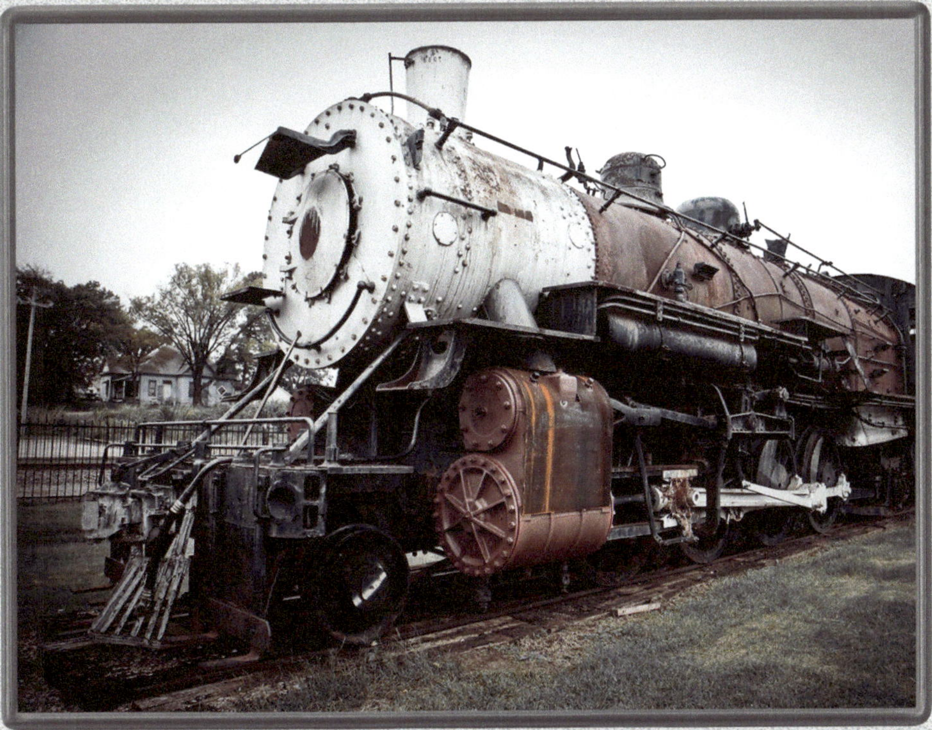

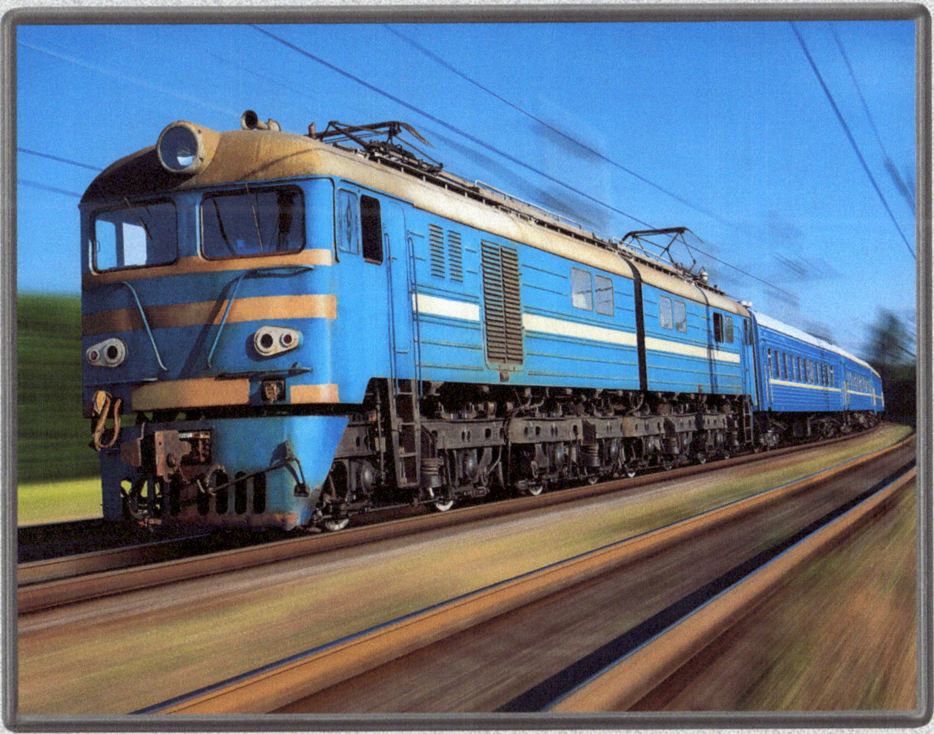

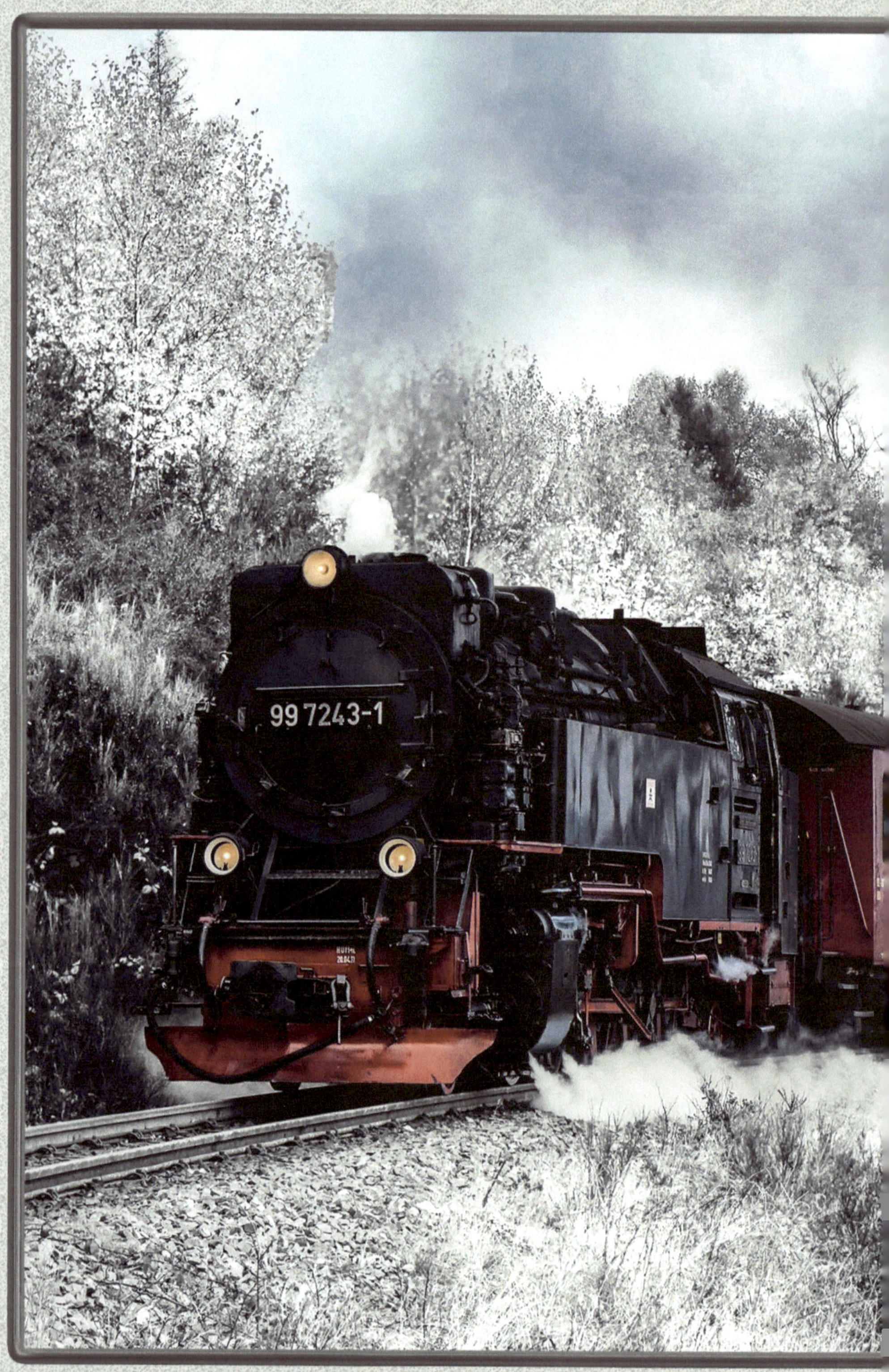

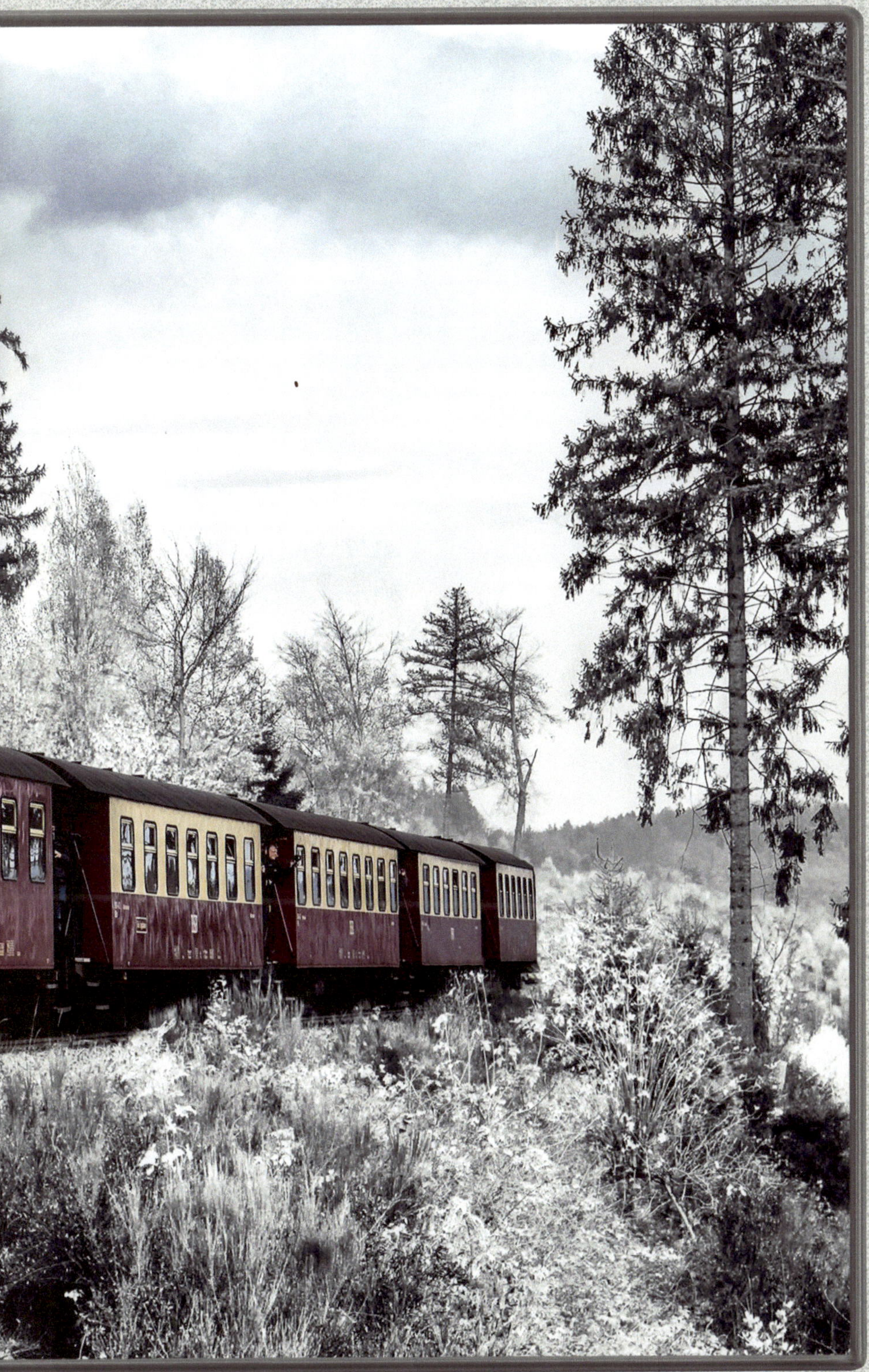

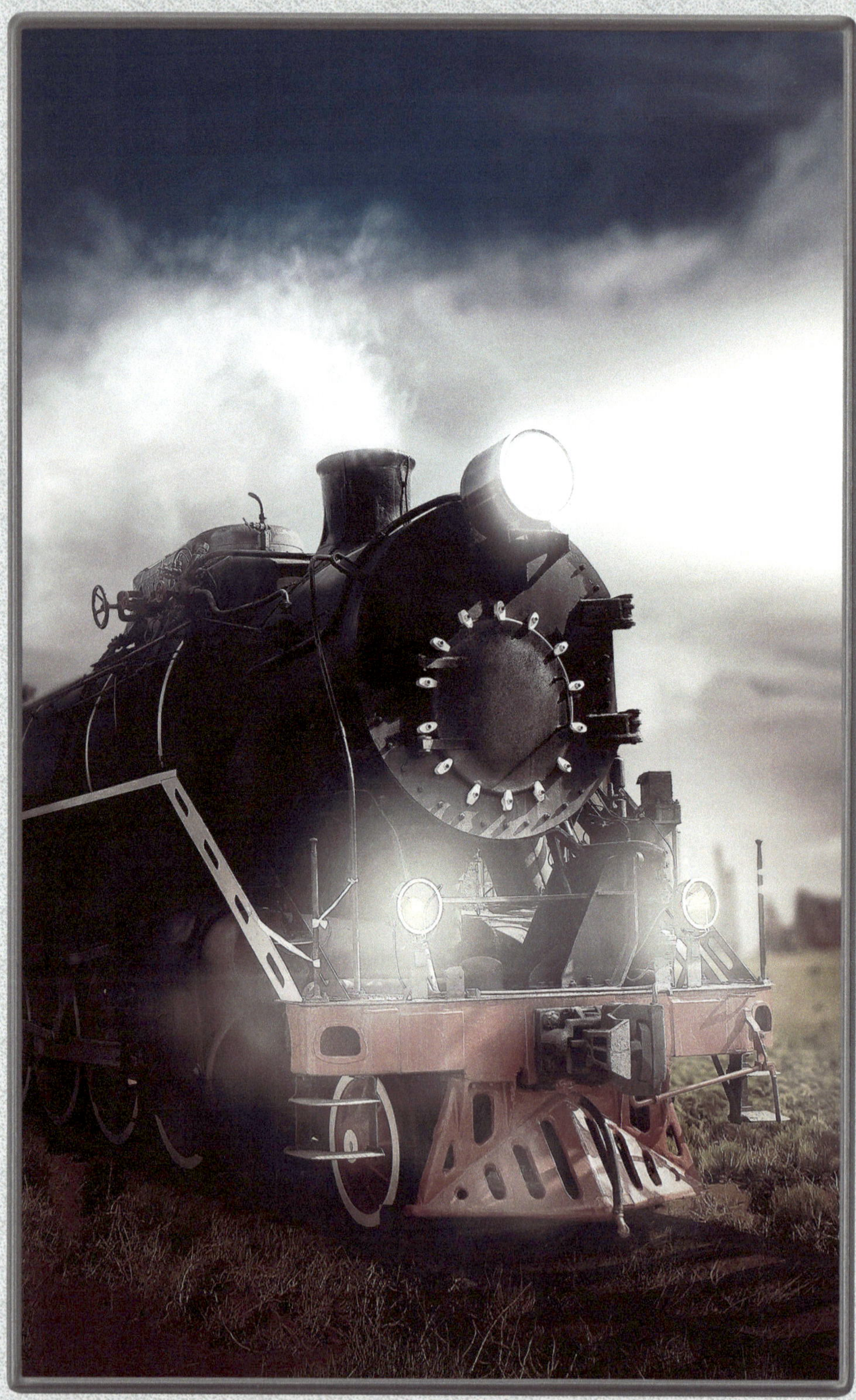

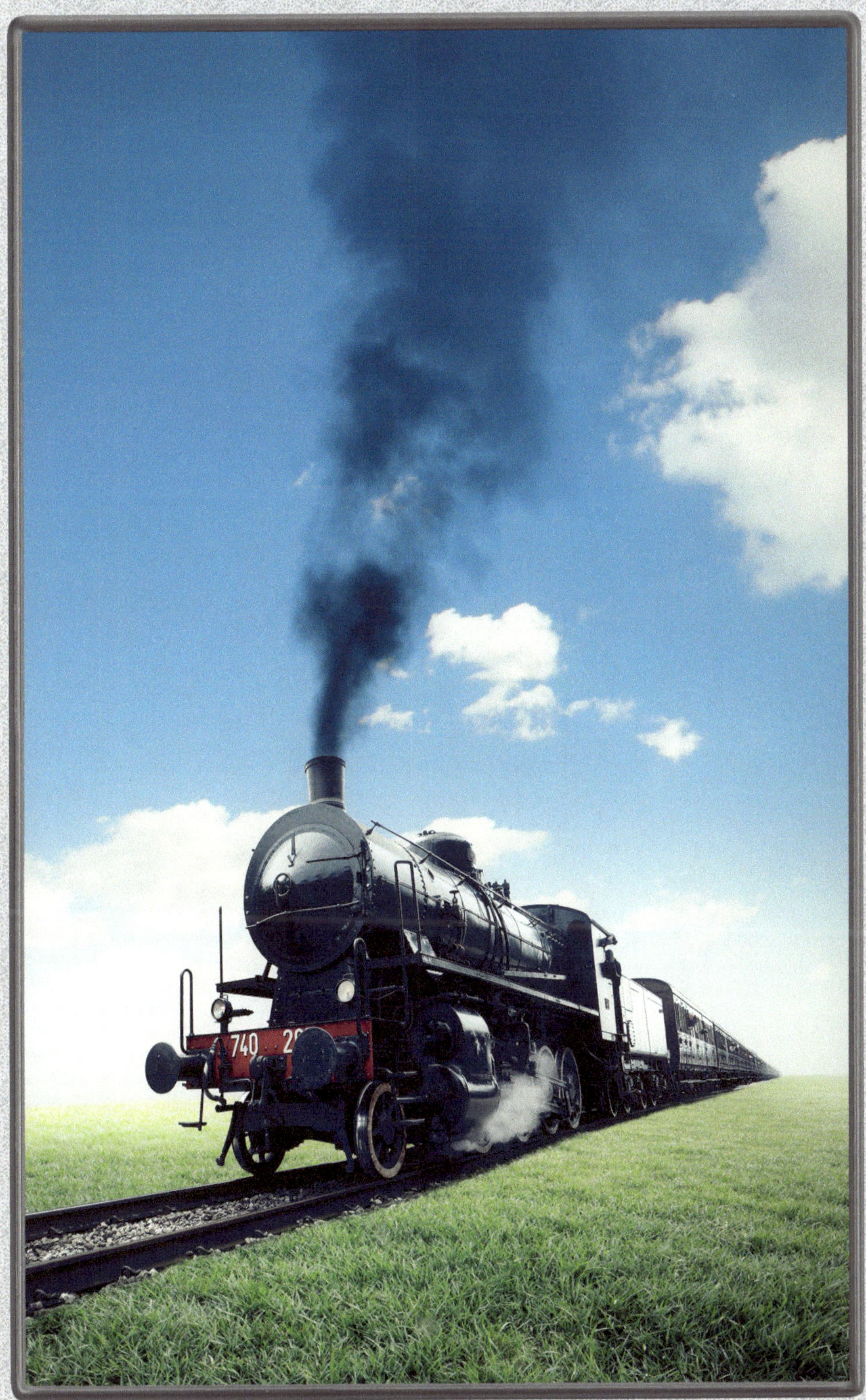
740   2

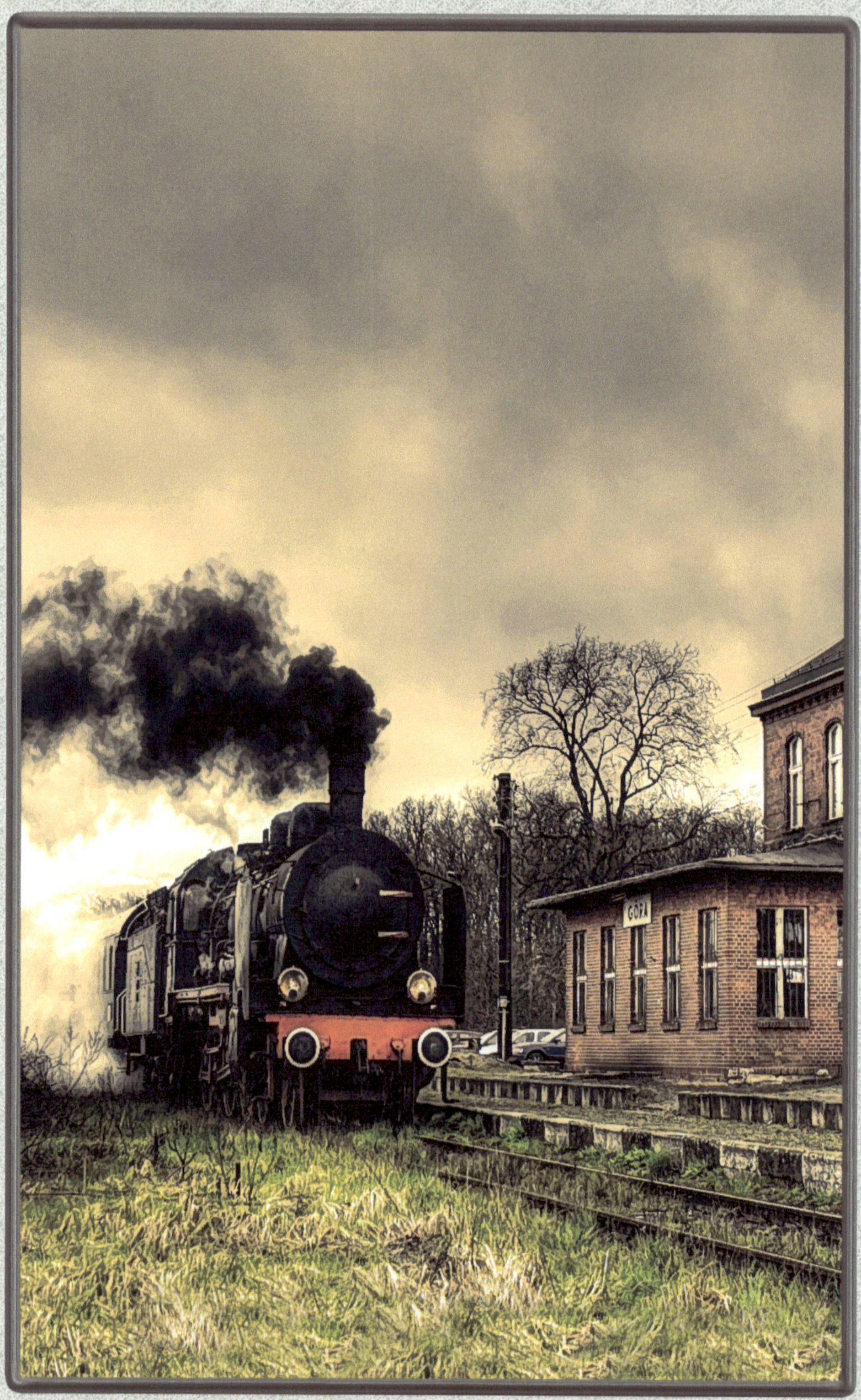
GÓRA

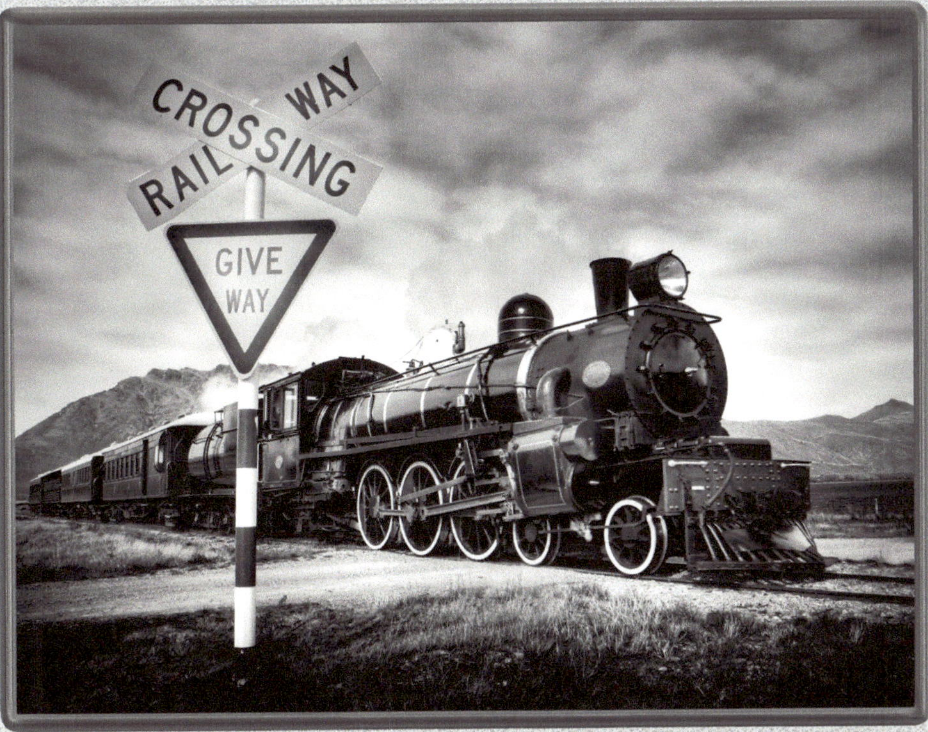

WAY
CROSSING
RAIL
GIVE
WAY

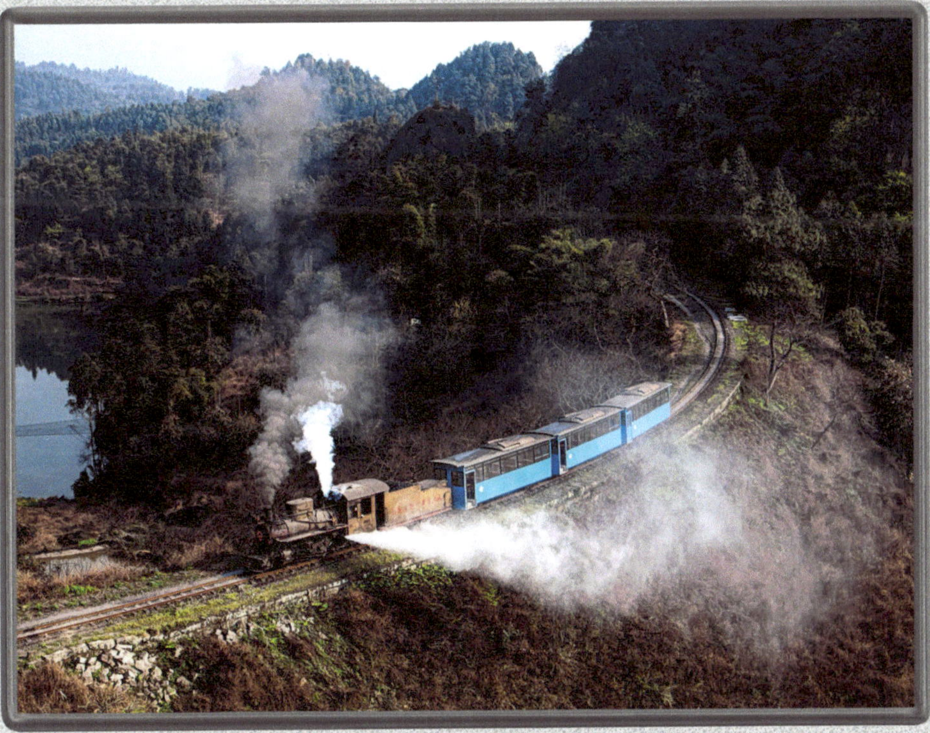

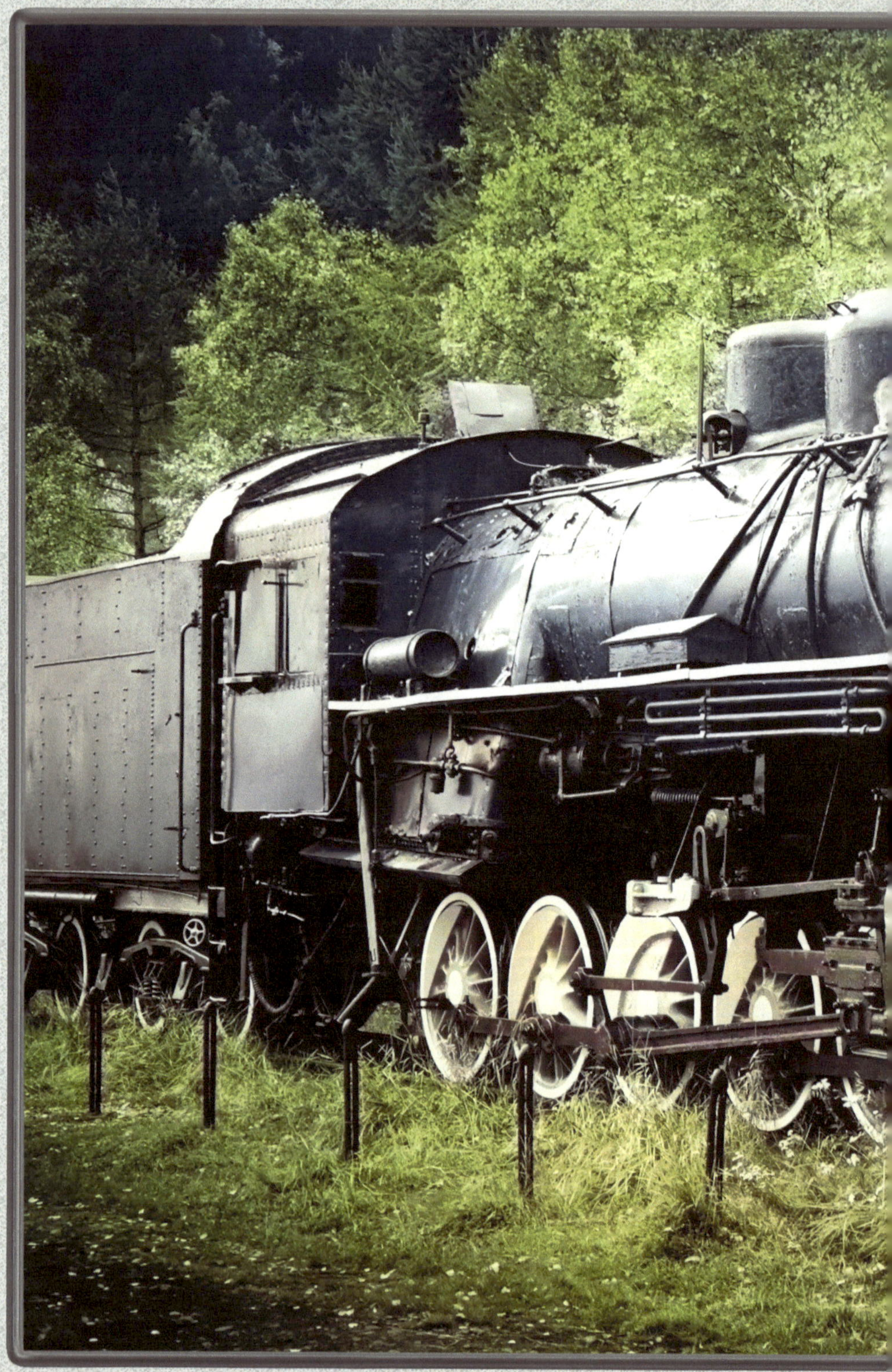

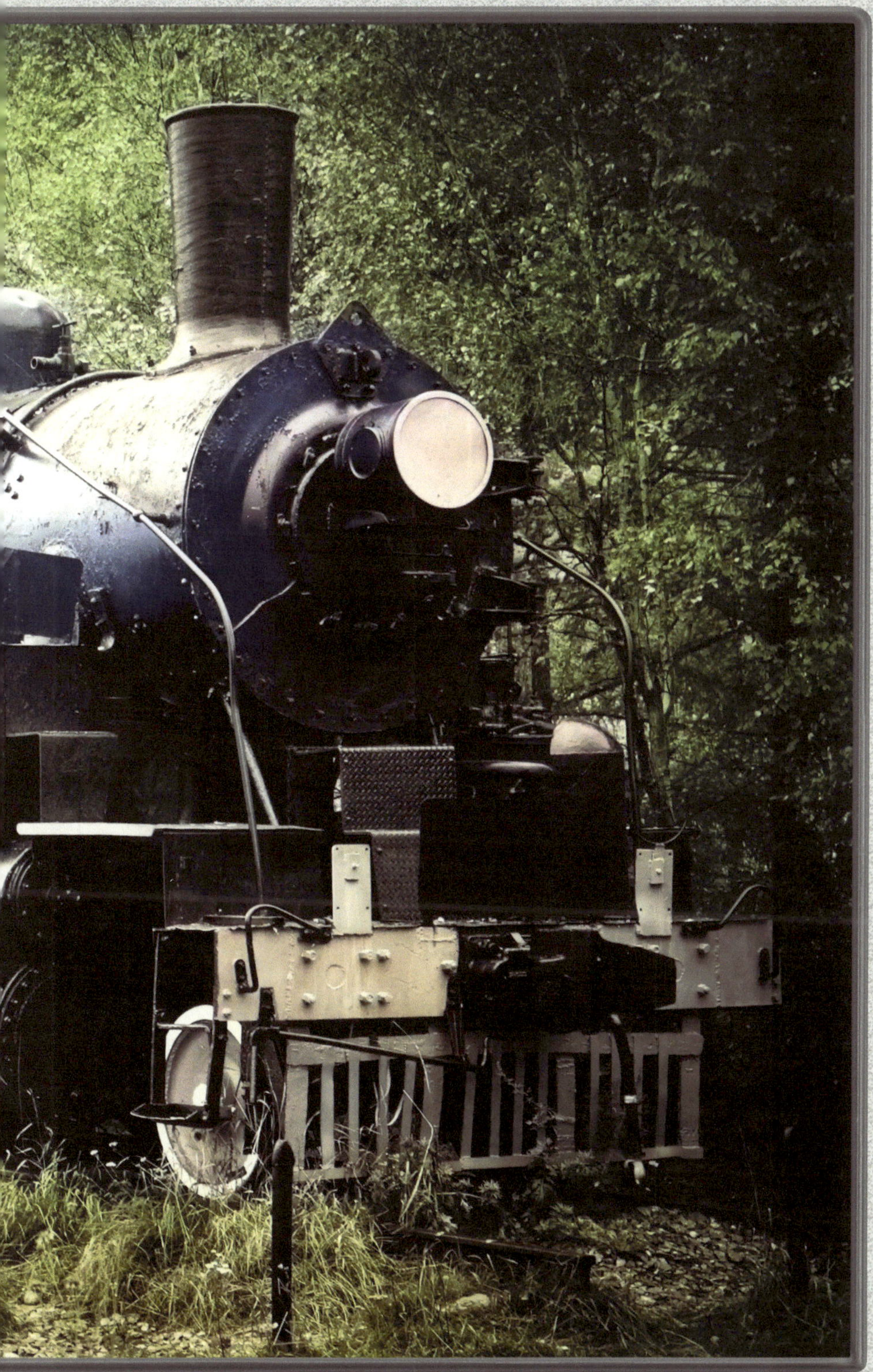

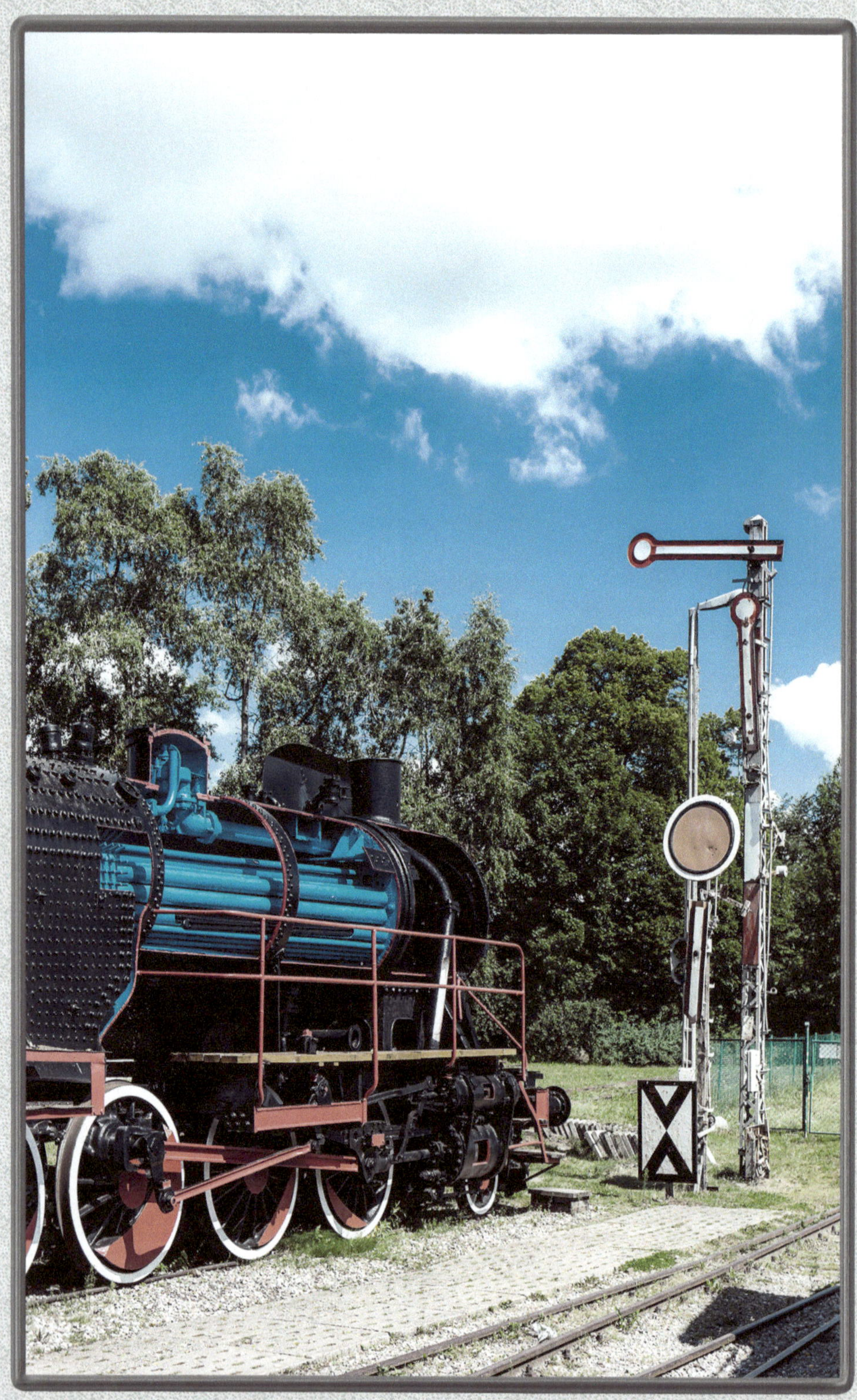

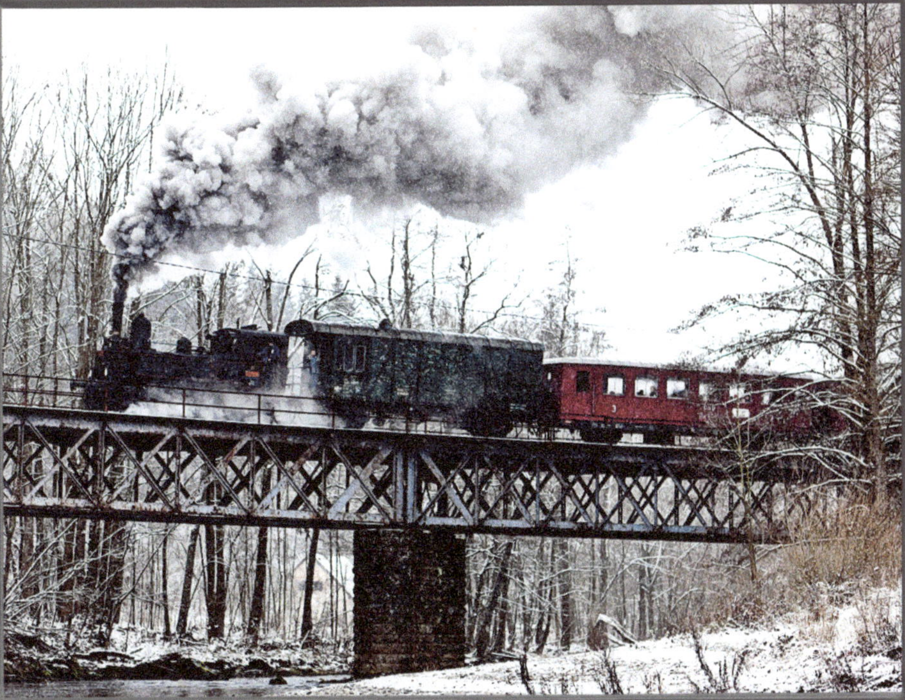

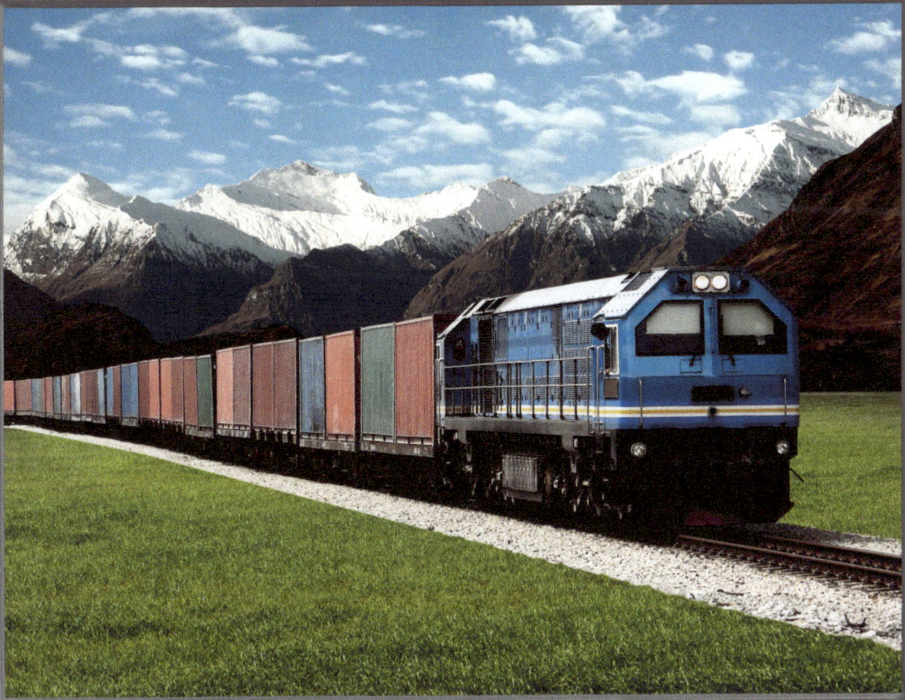

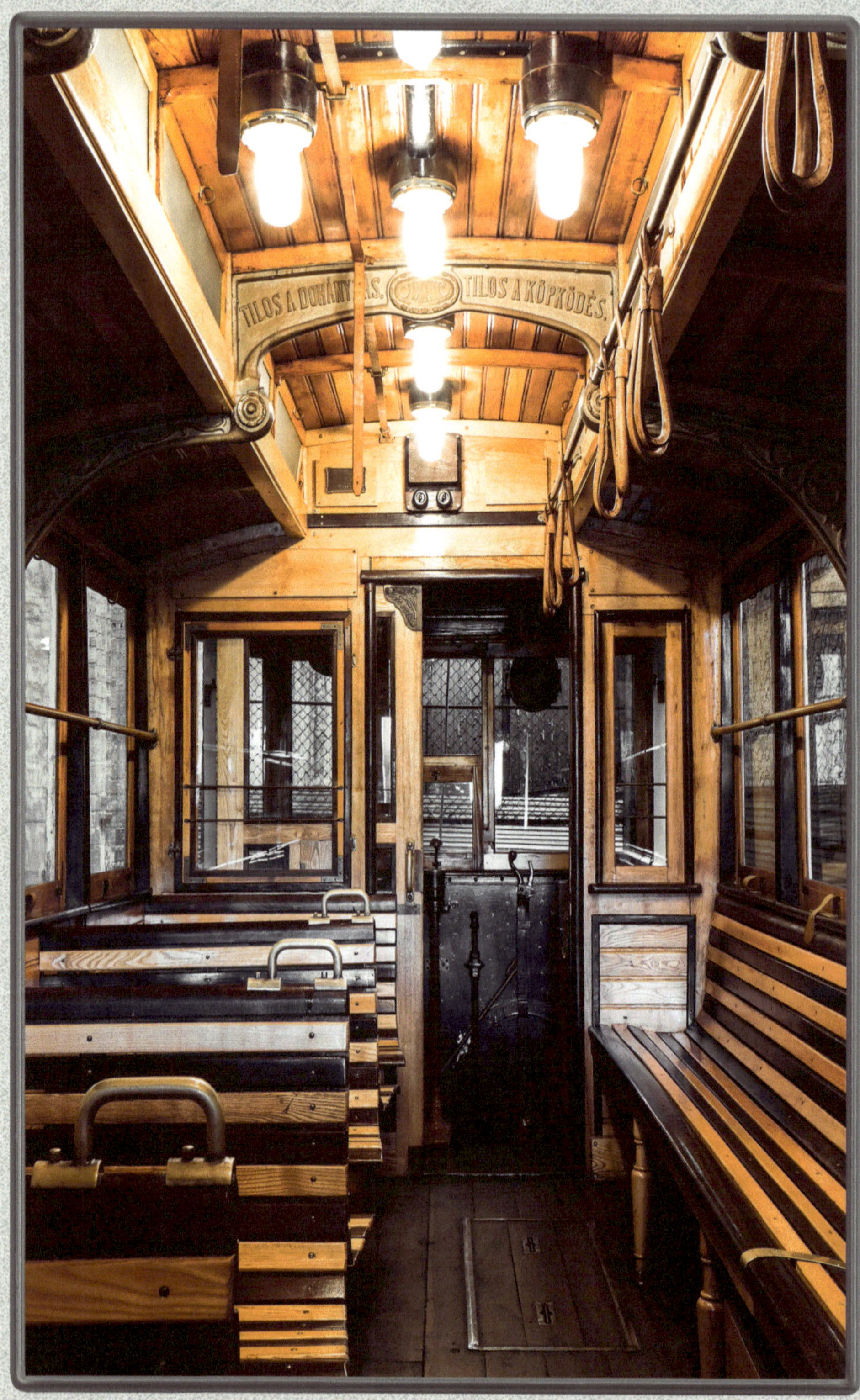

TILOS A DOHÁNYZÁS.
TILOS A KÖPKÖDÉS.

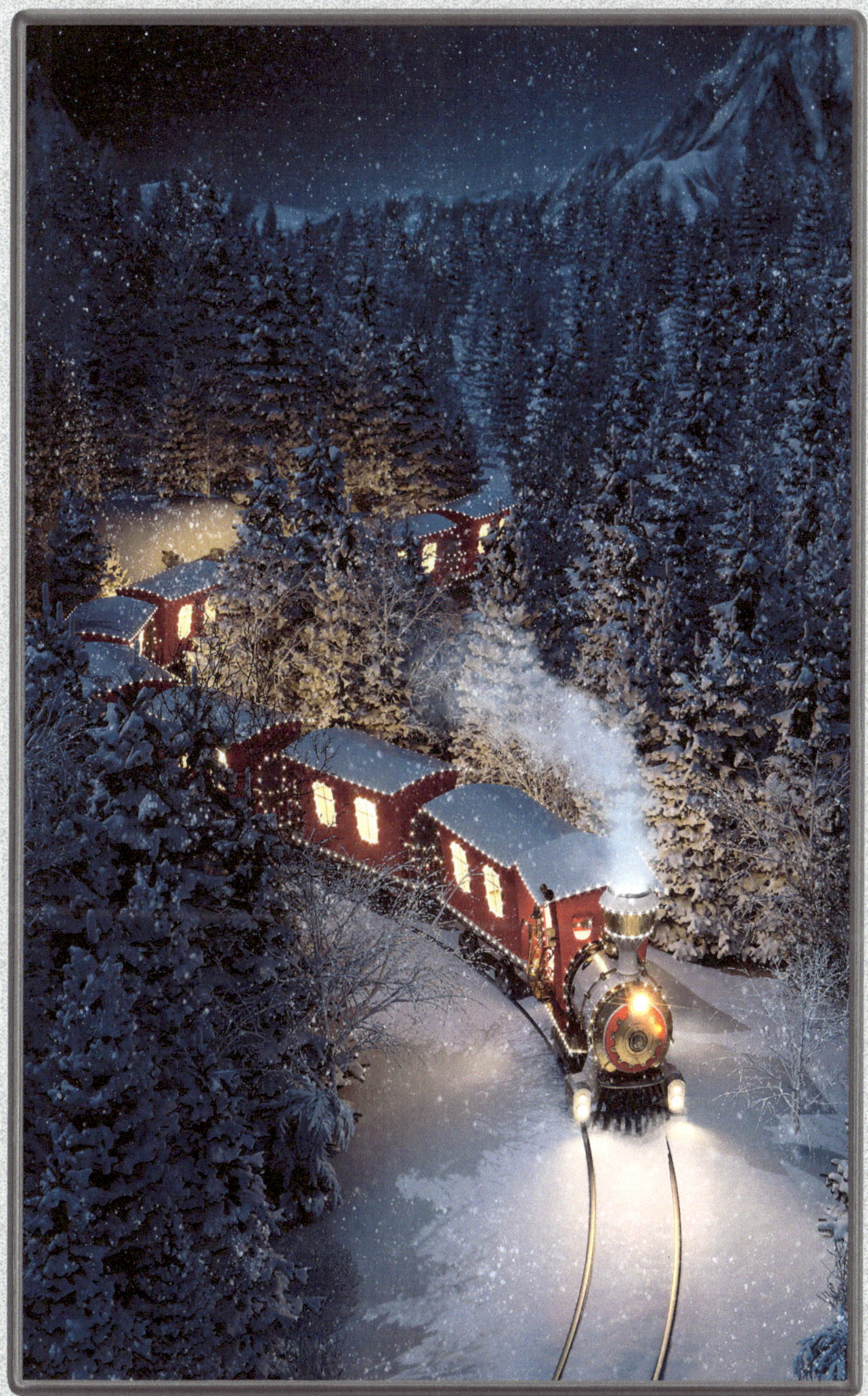